GETTING THINGS DONE

STOP BEING SO LAZY!

How Decluttering and Life Organization Can Lead You To Greater Productivity, Emotional Control, Self-Discipline, and True Happiness

GREYSON CAMERON

Copyright © 2020 Greyson Cameron

All Rights Reserved

Copyright 2020 By Greyson Cameron - All rights reserved.

The following book is produced below with the goal of providing information that is as accurate and reliable as possible. Regardless, purchasing this eBook can be seen as consent to the fact that both the publisher and the author of this book are in no way experts on the topics discussed within and that any recommendations or suggestions that are made herein are for entertainment purposes only. Professionals should be consulted as needed prior to undertaking any of the action endorsed herein.

This declaration is deemed fair and valid by both the American Bar Association and the Committee of Publishers Association and is legally binding throughout the United States.

Furthermore, the transmission, duplication or reproduction of any of the following work including specific information will be considered an illegal act irrespective of if it is done electronically or in print. This extends to creating a secondary or tertiary copy of the work or a recorded copy and is only allowed with express written consent from the Publisher. All additional right reserved.

The information in the following pages is broadly considered to be a truthful and accurate account of facts and as such any inattention, use or misuse of the information in question by the reader will render any resulting actions solely under their purview. There are no scenarios in which the publisher or the original author of this work can be in any fashion deemed liable for any hardship or damages that may befall them after undertaking information described herein.

Additionally, the information in the following pages is intended only for informational purposes and should thus be thought of as universal. As befitting its nature, it is presented without assurance regarding its prolonged validity or interim quality. Trademarks that are mentioned are done without written consent and can in no way be considered an endorsement from the trademark holder.

Table of Contents

PART I 11

Chapter 1: What is Holding You Back 12

Why People Procrastinate 12

- Abstract Goals 14
- Not Having Foreseeable Rewards 15
- A Disconnect from Our Future Selves 15
- Being Too Optimistic 16
- Being Indecisive 17
- Task Aversion 17
- Perfectionism 18
- Self-Handicapping 18

Other Major Reasons for Not Getting Things Done 19

- Not Sure What to do 20
- There is No Deadline or Accountability 20
- Don't See Any Consequences 21

Why Getting Things Done is Critical 21

Chapter 2: It's Time to Get Things Done 24

Overcoming Procrastination 24

- Don't Catastrophize 24
- Focus on Your "Why" 25
- Get Out Your Scheduler 25
- Be Realistic 26
- Break it Down 26
- Stop With the Excuses 27

- Find an Accountability Partner 27
- Optimize Your Environment 27
- Forgive Yourself 28
- **Mindfulness Meditation Technique** 28
  - Body Scan Meditation 29
  - Sitting Meditation 29
  - Walking Meditation 29
  - Simple Mindfulness 30
- **15 Habits of Highly Productive People** 30

Chapter 3: Visualizing a Better Future 33

- **How to Visualize Your Future** 33
- **More Tips for Visualization** 34
  - Visualize Your New Life 34
  - Create a Vision Board 35
  - Write Down Your goals 35
  - Let Yourself Zone Out 35
  - Say Your Goals Out Loud 36
  - Think About What You Want and not What You Don't Want 36
- **Life When You Get Things Done** 36
  - A Feeling of Relaxed Control 37
  - Your Thinking Will Be Stimulated 37
  - More Organization and Less Clutter 37
  - Less Time for Worry 38

PART II 40

Chapter 1: The Clutter in Your Life 41

- **Why You Have Clutter** 42
  - You Don't Recognize What Clutter Is 42

You Don't Know How Long You Should Keep Something.................43
You Don't Know How to Store Things.................................43
You Are Not Using Clutter Busters 44
Buying Too Many Things, You Don't Need............................44
You Can't Let Things Go 45

Endowment Effect 45
The Consequences of Too Much Clutter 46

Your Stress Levels Increase..47
Your Diet Is Impacted in A Negative Way...............................47
You Can Develop More Respiratory Issues..............................47
Your Safety Is Threatened 48
Your Love Life Is Jeopardized 48
Your Kids Will Be Upset 49
You Will Become Isolated 49
You Will Miss Out On Getting Promoted 49
You Are More Likely to Miss Work......................................50
Your Productivity Decreases...50
You Will Develop Poor Spending Habits................................51
You Can Go into Debt..51

Clutter is Not Just Physical...52
Chapter 2: Breaking Your Relationship With "Stuff" 54

Getting Over the Endowment Effect....................................54
More Decluttering Tips...55
Stop Buying Stuff You Don't Need 57
The Benefits Of Decluttering 60
Decluttering Equals Increased Focus and Productivity 61
Decluttering and Improved Health 62

Improved Healthy Habits 62

Better Self-Care 63

Losing Weight 63

Easier to Relax 64

Having More Space 64

6-Week Decluttering Challenge 65

Chapter 1: Is This for You? 69

Chapter 2: Your Toolbox, DBT 71

Chapter 3: Finding Yourself through Mindfulness 76

Chapter 4: Taking Mindfulness to the Next Level with Advanced Meditation Techniques 80

Chapter 5: Using Your New Tools to Process Negative Emotions 85

Chapter 6: Defining Your Goals, Your Values, and Yourself 89

Chapter 7: Living in the Positive! 92

Chapter 8: How DBT Has Enhanced Your Life 96

Chapter 1: Self-Care Is the Best Care 147

How Does Self-Care Work 148

How Does Self-Care Improve Self-Esteem and Self-Confidence? 149

Chapter 2: 152

What Does Good Self-Care Look Like? 152

Good Self-Care Practices 152

Taking Responsibility for Your Happiness 152

You Become Assertive With Others 152

You Treat Yourself As You Would a Close Friend 152

You Are Not Afraid to Ask for What You Want 153

Your Life Is Set Around Your Own Values 153

Chapter 3: Demanding Your Own Self-Care 154

Setting Healthy Boundaries 154

Identify and Name Your Limits 154

Stay Tuned Into Your Feelings 155

Don't Be Afraid of Being Direct 155

Give Yourself Permission to Set Boundaries 155

Consider Your Past and Present 156

Be Assertive 156

Start Small 156

Eliminating Toxicity and Not Caring About Losing Friends 157

Don't Expect People to Change 157

Establish and Maintain Boundaries 157

Don't Keep Falling for Crisis Situations 157

Focus on the Solution 158

Accept Your Own Difficulties and Weaknesses 158

They Won't Go Easily 158

Choose Your Battles Carefully 159

Surround Yourself With Healthy relationships 159

How to Focus on Self-Care 159

Pay Attention to Your Sleep 159

Take Care of Your Gut 160

Exercise and Physical Activity Is Essential 160

Consider a Mediterranean Diet 160

Take a Self-Care Trip 161

Get Outside 161

Bring a Pet Into Your Life 161

- Get Yourself Organized 161
- Cook Yourself Meals At Home 161
- Read Regularly 162
- Schedule Your Self-Care Time 162

Chapter 4: How to Be Happy Being Alone 163

- **Accept Some Alone Time** 163
  - Do Not Compare Yourself to Others 163
  - Step Away From Social Media 163
  - Take a Break From Your Phone 164
  - Allow Time for Your Mind to Wander 164
  - Take Yourself on a Date 164
  - Exercise 164
  - Take Advantage of the Perks of Being Alone 164
  - Find a Creative Outlet 165
  - Take Time to Self-Reflect 165
  - Make Plans for Your Future 165
  - Make Plans for Solo Outings 165

PART I

Chapter 1: What is Holding You Back

The first half of this book focused on the negative aspects of clutter and how removing unnecessary items from your life can be cathartic in so many ways. The goal of all of this was to begin getting things done in your life. This includes all aspects of a person's personal and professional life. Honestly, decluttering was just the first step. It was a way to clear up our minds and reduce distractions. After doing this, it is time to start moving forward and getting things done in our lives. Now that our physical and mental spaces are clear, what else can we focus on? The goal of this chapter is to present some of the biggest challenges to getting things done.

Why People Procrastinate

Procrastination is something many people in our society suffer with. It is the purposeful and unnecessary delay of actions or decisions. Why do something now when you can just do it tomorrow? Well, because you never know what tomorrow will bring. Other challenges will arise, distractions will come up, and you will continue to load up your plate because you refuse to take things off of it. Since you are making the excuse today for waiting until tomorrow, what is stopping you from making the same excuse tomorrow, or the next day and the next day?

Imagine being at a buffet and loading up your plate. When you go to sit down, you decide not to eat much of the food because you want it later. Instead, you go and grab another plate to fill up and bring back to the table. Now, you have two plates to finish, and you have no idea how you will do it. Eventually, the restaurant is about to close, and you don't have the time or space to finish everything. You will most likely waste a large portion of the food. This is what procrastination looks like in life. You keep pushing things back until you become overloaded, overwhelmed, and very close to the deadline, if you even make it at all.

Procrastination is one of the worst enemies of getting things done. It really has no value, except for the fact that some people thrive on making quick deadlines. However, you will also be more likely to make big mistakes. You will never be able to complete the work to your full potential because so many things will be missed. Even if they're minor, they still add up.

Procrastination leads to so many missed opportunities too. Several people do not pursue their goals because they put them off for too long. Eventually, they get to the point where they lose interest or become too involved in other things to where they no longer have time.

People assume that procrastination has everything to do with will power. While this can be a major reason, for sure, it is not the only one that exists. There are many deeper reasons for why people put things off. There are some psychological aspects that are at play. For example, anxiety and fear of failure will terrify people into paralysis. Nobody wants to fail, and if they start something, failure is a huge possibility. As a result, we delay starting anything. At least then, we can save face a little bit.

When our motivation to complete a task outweighs the negative aspects, then there's a strong chance we will still finish it. However, if the negative aspects outweigh our own motivation, then we will put off pursuing a goal if we even do so at all. The following are some other factors that keep up from moving forward. If we follow these, we will always procrastinate.

Abstract Goals

If a person has a vague or abstract goal, then they are more likely to procrastinate. They are not excited enough about it. In fact, they might not even know what the goal is, as there is no clear definition. For example, making a promise to get fit is an abstract goal. It is a simple statement with no real substance. What are the chances you will get fit if you have no actual plan in place for doing so? Furthermore, what does "get fit" even mean to? Does it mean losing a certain amount of weight, gaining muscle, looking slimmer, having more energy, or a combination of all? Honestly, you are not even giving yourself a chance to obtain this goal, as you will just put it off until you forget about it.

A more solid goal would be, "I will lose 15 pounds within two months and be able to run six miles by then." This is a concrete goal with real values and end results. From here, you can create specific action steps to get there. For example, losing two pounds and increasing your run mileage by one every week. Once you create real goals with a legitimate plan, then you are more likely to not put things off.

Not Having Foreseeable Rewards

Many individuals put things off because they see no actual rewards in the near future. For example, a teenager may not attend college because he or she cannot fathom waiting four years or more to get a degree in something that might make them money. In addition, the money will not come right away, which is another deterrent.

People often want immediate pleasure rather than long-term success. This can be seen in people neglecting to create savings or investment accounts. They do not want money later; they want it now. As a result, they delay setting up one of these essential accounts because they can't see the benefits they will create in the future.

This same mindset can apply to punishments, as well. The farther into the future a punishment is, the less likely it will motivate someone to take action. If you are studying for a final exam in college and it is months away, you are not that concerned about it, because even if you fail, it will be a while until that actually happens.

A Disconnect from Our Future Selves

People tend to procrastinate because they cannot comprehend a connection between their present and future selves. They believe the two individuals are mutually exclusive for some reason and don't realize that they are creating their future person by the actions you take today.

A person may delay starting a healthy diet because they cannot see themselves overweight and dealing with chronic diseases in the future. A company someone works for has a chance of going out of business, but the employee does not work on his resume because he cannot see himself being out of work. In both of these examples, their present and future selves are completely different people.

Being Too Optimistic

Now, being optimistic is not a bad thing; however, getting to the point where you overthink your abilities can be a problem. This is a common occurrence as many people do not work on tasks in the present because they highly believe they can complete it in the future. While this may be true, there will still be an increased amount of stress and anxiety. Also, the potential for oversight and significant errors will be present.

Imagine that you have a 10,000-word paper due to Friday, and it is only Monday. It would make sense to write 1,000-2,000 words daily, instead of waiting until Wednesday or Thursday. When writing the paper ahead of time, you will have extra opportunities to think everything through, and also go back and edit your work. Giving yourself extra time will help you in creating quality work.

Being Indecisive

This is when you cannot make a move because you cannot decide what course of action to take. For example, you may hesitate to apply for a job because you cannot decide which one is best for you. This is a phenomenon known as analysis paralysis, and it has stopped many great people right in their tracks. The following are some factors that make it difficult to make a decision.

- The more options you have, the harder it will be to decide a preferable path to take.
- The more similar different options are, the harder it will be to choose. You might end up analyzing the smallest sectors of each choice.
- The more important the decision is, the harder it will be to make because of the impact it will have on you and others.

It is best if you can keep your decisions to a minimum, as well as your choices. Each time you make a decision, you deplete your mental resources to a degree. So, if you make a host of decisions in a short time period, you have a high likelihood of getting burned out.

Task Aversion

People often procrastinate because they are not looking forward to a task they need to perform. For example, they might have to call them back to resolve a payment dispute but are not looking forward to talking with a customer service representative. As a result, They put off doing it. If you are avoiding a task because of the aversion you have to it, you are just delaying your agony. Imagine how good you will feel after doing it. So, hold your nose and get it done.

Perfectionism

People often want things so perfect that they are terrified of doing something out of fear of the mistakes they will make. Instead of starting and taking their chances, they avoid moving forward. Perfectionism has been called the enemy of productivity because of all the delays it creates along the way. People do not realize that things will no be perfect, so they waste excessive time trying to ake things this way.

Self-Handicapping

Many individuals are terrified of exposing their lack of ability for something. As a result, they procrastinate so they can use it as an excuse for poor performance. They would rather that people think they're lazy than incapable. Procrastinators with this mindset are more likely to put things off if they feel that failure will reflect badly on them.

These are some of the most common reasons for procrastination. There is no easy answer to why people avoid doing things, but it must be overcome for people to start accomplishing things. The following are a few more reasons for procrastination:

- Self-sabotage
- Low self-efficacy
- Perceived lack of self-control
- Fear of being criticized

Sometimes, there are more urgent situations, like ADHD, depression, or low self-esteem, that need to be addressed. The better question to ask is: Why put something off until tomorrow if I can get it done today?

Other Major Reasons for Not Getting Things Done

For some reason, people are just not getting as many things done as they could. Now, I am not saying you have to be on the go all the time. That is not healthy, either. What I am saying is that you need to accomplish things within a certain time period, or you will never achieve anything in life. This will not just affect you, but those who rely on you, as well, like employees, business partners, and family members. To make the world go around, people need to get things done. Yet, they don't. I already spoke about procrastination as a major factor. I will now detail a few other reasons why this happens.

Not Sure What to do

Many people do not do anything because they have no idea what they should do. Even if they have a goal, they are clueless about how to get started in any way. This often occurs because we see other people's accomplishments but have no idea how they achieved them. We keep trying to guess but can't figure it out. Even if we do become aware of how something was accomplished, the values do not line up with our own, which makes us even more confused. It is better to keep on track with your own beliefs when trying to accomplish a goal, rather than rejecting them completely. Rejecting your values will make you even more confused.

There is No Deadline or Accountability

Accountability seems to be going by the wayside these days. People don't get things done because they are not expected to. There is often no disciplinary actions taken, so people continue to lack the drive to move forwards.

Also, when deadlines are nonexistent, then there is no need to get moving. Either we don't create deadlines for ourselves, or other people don't place them on us. If you work for someone and they do not set deadlines, then the operations of the company are not very sound. If you do not set your own deadlines for goals, then you need to start doing so. Make them concrete and not too far out. Remember, you don't want to fall into a procrastination step.

Set a specific date for when you want to accomplish something and stick to it completely. Set it around important events if you can. For example, if you are planning a vacation or will be attending a concert, make it a goal to finish a certain project or reach a specific endpoint. If you are attending a wedding, and you also need to get in shape to fit into your suit, you can make a goal to lose 10 pounds prior to the wedding.

Don't See Any Consequences

This goes along the lines of accountability, but the reason so many people don't get things done is that they do not realize the consequences until they already occur. For example, if your roof needs to be fixed, you will probably put it off because you do not see any consequences for doing so. Of course, on the night that it's pouring rain and the roof suddenly collapses, you will recognize your mistake. Start seeing the potential consequences of not getting things done. Write them down if you have to. Once you see them visually, then you are more likely to take them seriously. For example, if you need new tires on your car and you have been putting it off, then write down that you will get stranded on the freeway with four ruptured tires.

Why Getting Things Done is Critical

Here is the bottom line. The many advancements we have made in this world were done by go-getters who acted constantly. They were not done by people who refused to do the work. As you look back on history, any type of accomplishment, whether good or bad, had massive action behind it. I say bad, as well, because there have been many negative events in our history. I hope you keep your goals positive.

Getting things done creates a sense of accomplishment. No matter how much or how little you do today, it is far better than doing nothing. Nothing gets you nowhere while small steps create some progress.

Getting things done now is the ultimate productivity hack available. There are no tricks or secret formulas. It is simply a matter of doing something now, rather than nothing at all. Whatever you can manage to do within a given period of time, do it, and you will be that much closer.

Imagine having to paint a house. This is not an easy task, especially if you have a big house. Let's say, for this example, the house has 100 walls to paint. If you pain one a day, that is still something. After 100 days, which is just over three months, you will have painted the whole house. Taking three months is better than nothing at all. On certain days, when you have more time and energy, you can paint extra on those days. If painting your house is a goal, then give yourself a deadline with rewards or punishments along the way. For example, if you are not halfway done by a certain date, then cancel something you were looking forward to. Hold yourself accountable, and if you need to, have someone else hold you accountable too.

In the next chapter, I will cover many different tips to start getting things done.

Chapter 2: It's Time to Get Things Done

Now that I have covered the reason why people don't get things done; it is now time to start taking action. This chapter will be focused on various strategies to overcome the blocks in your life. Start following these, and you will be accomplishing things in no time.

Overcoming Procrastination

It's time to stop putting things off. Many of your dreams and goals have gone unfulfilled because you waited too long to start working on them. The world has also missed out on your gifts because you had the potential to create something great if you only took some action in completing it. The following are some ways to overcome one of the greatest obstacles to not getting something done: Procrastination.

Don't Catastrophize

This means that you make a bigger deal out of things than you should. This could be based on the results you might get, or the excruciating the actual task will be. In any event, you are expecting the process to be unbearable.

Here's a little tip: it won't be. We often overthink to the point that our mind creates a scenario that is not conducive to reality. The truth is, hard work, boredom, and other challenges will not kill you. You may not enjoy them on time, but you will overcome them. Also, the results we get are rarely ever at the level we imagine them to be. The thought of a fall is generally harder than the fall itself.

Always believe in yourself that you can make it through something and deal with the consequences, positive or negative, that come with it. The truth is, you can. Even if a task is as horrible as you imagined, you got through it, and it's out of the way. This is much better than thinking about it. Just get it done!

Focus on Your "Why"

You "why" is the ultimate reason for you doing something and should be used as a motivating factor for you. Many procrastinators focus on short-term gains and do not pay attention to long-term potential. This is why it's important to remember your "why." It is the end result you are expecting.

This can be used for any goal in your life, personal or professional. If you have been putting off creating a resume, then imagine yourself in your dream job. If you have been putting off organizing your room, imagine how good you will feel when you can find things easily and don't have to get around a huge mess.

Get Out Your Scheduler

Projects often do not get done because people make no time for them. They will do it when they have time, and therefore, the time will never come. You need to make time and stick to it. Get out your scheduler, whether it's an online planner, paper planner, or calendar, and start blocking off times. Whatever important tasks that need to be completed, write them down and on a specific time and date. Unless something unavoidable comes up, stick to the specific block on your schedule. When people write things down, they are holding themselves accountable. If they miss doing something, they can look at it, and it will remind them.

Be Realistic

Getting things done means you are setting yourself up for success. Do not create unrealistic goals for yourself. Set an achievable goal, and then take specific action steps to get there. For example, do not tell yourself that you will start working out five times a week in the morning immediately when you are not even a morning person. Instead, set up your workout schedule in the evening. If you ultimately want to work out in the mornings, then you can start by doing it once a week and then increasing your days. Do not expect to reach your goals instantly. Set up a long-term plan for success

Break it Down

Tasks can often become overwhelming, and this leads to procrastination. Break them down into smaller and more manageable tasks with specific deadlines for each small task. If you are planning to landscape your home, start with a small area and give yourself the time you need in each section.

Stop With the Excuses

Here it goes: You will never be fully energized; it will never be the right time; you will often not be in the mood; conditions may never be perfect. Stop using these as excuses. Waiting for any of these will just delay you for no reason. Getting things done is not about waiting for the perfect opportunity. It is about using what you ave to create opportunity. Stop with the excuses!

Find an Accountability Partner

It can be difficult to hold yourself accountable, so find a partner to help you. Express what your goals are to this person and the deadlines that you have. Your accountability partner can then follow up with you and make sure you are staying on track. If you don't reach your deadlines, your partner's job is to grill you as to why. You guys can help each other in this manner to make it a mutual relationship.

Optimize Your Environment

Your environment will play a huge role in creating distractions. Optimize it by finding a quiet place and only having the things you absolutely need. Turn off the TV, social media (I recommend logging out so you can't access it easily), get rid of any papers or clutter that will catch your attention. How many times have you meant to start something, only to get distracted by something else? This is very common, and you must do what you can to avoid it happening to you.

Forgive Yourself

While it might be true that starting something earlier would have been more advantageous, do not beat yourself up for not doing so. You cannot change the past, so forget about it. You can make up for it though by taking advantage of the present. Learn from your past mistake of putting something off and start doing things today. If you should have gone to college five years ago, well, it's okay. You can still go now.

Procrastinators are often trying to avoid distress, but in doing so, they are ironically creating more of it. Start taking the action steps I have described above, and you will no longer be putting things off until tomorrow.

Mindfulness Meditation Technique

Many individuals are not able to get things done because they cannot live in the present moment. They are either anxious about the past or worried about the future. Both of these are unproductive thoughts to have and must be eliminated immediately. You must start focusing on the present, and mindfulness meditation techniques are a great way to do so. Bear in mind, it can take years to master the practice of meditation, so I will just go over the basics to get you started. The following are some structured meditation exercises.

Body Scan Meditation

Start by lying down on your back with your arms at your sides, palms facing up, and legs extended. Now pay close attention and observe every section of your body from head to toe. Become fully aware of any sensations or emotions you are feeling and from where they are coming from. This will bring awareness to yourself and what is happening to you. You will begin living in the present moment with real-time feelings.

Sitting Meditation

Sit in a comfortable position, preferable in a chair, with your back straight, feet flat on the floor, and your palms on your lap. Once in a comfortable position, breathe in slowly through your nose and allow it to go down to your diaphragm. Then slowly let the breath out. Focus completely on your breathing. If you get distracted by anything, note the experience and then return your attention back to your breathing.

Walking Meditation

Find a quiet space that is at least 15-20 feet in length. Walk slowly between each wall in the room and focus completely on the experience. Be aware of all of the subtle movements that are being used to keep you balanced. Do not pay attention to anything else but your walking.

Simple Mindfulness

The following are a few more mindfulness exercises. These are simple and can be practiced anywhere.

- Focus on your breathing. Take slow and deep breaths in and out. This was done in the meditative position but can also be accomplished standing up anywhere.
- Find joy in the simple pleasures of life and live in the moment.
- Accept yourself and learn to treat yourself like you would a good friend.
- Experience the environment you are in with all of your senses. Do not be in such a rush all the time. Fully taste the food you're eating, stop to smell the roses, listen to the birds chirping, and even touch some dirt. Feel your surroundings.

15 Habits of Highly Productive People

To become successful, you must mimic the habits of other successful people. The following are effective habits that productive people use every day. These individuals get things done, and you can, as well.

- Focus on the most important tasks first. These are the ones that have the most urgency, the closest deadlines, and the most with the most severe results if not done. Complete them first and then move on to other things.
- Cultivate deep work, which are your hardest, most boring, and most complicated tasks. They have to be done, and if you are not focused fully, they will be missed. Say "no" to people more often, limit distractions, set up a scheduled time for these tasks each day, and go where you do your best work, whether in the office, library, or café, etc.
- Keep a distraction list. While you are working, anytime a distraction comes up, write it down, and then get back to work. This technique works because you are giving attention to your distraction, which eases up its strength over you.
- Use the 80/20 rule. Determine the 20% of your work that requires the most attention. Look at the remaining 80% and see what you can cut out to make more time for the 20%.
- Take scheduled breaks. Even though you want to get a lot done, you cannot just work 24/7. Take scheduled breaks throughout your workday and spend the rest of the time being fully focused. For instance, spend 55 minutes working hard, then take a 10 minutes break to relax and eat something.
- Limit the number of decisions you have to make. Decisions that aren't important should not take up too much of your time or energy. For example, many productive people will wear similar outfits every day because their wardrobe is not as important as other decisions.

- Eliminate insufficient communication. Ignore and delete useless emails, do not engage in too much idle chatter, and avoid gossip, which is a complete waste of time.
- Delegate certain tasks when you can. If you are busy with your career, then you can hire people to do things like take care of your lawn or do your dry cleaning.
- Learn from your successes, as well as your mistakes. Even in success, lessons can be learned about making things more efficient.
- Plan as much as you can for things going wrong because getting caught off guard can be quite a time consumer. It is better to have a plan ahead of time than trying to come up with one urgently.
- Don't wait until you are inspired or motivated to work. Start working and get yourself inspired or motivated.
- Avoid Multitasking. Instead, focus on one task for as long as you can before moving over to the next one.
- Get enough sleep, eat well, exercise, and take time to recharge. This will give you the energy you need when it's time to be productive. Whenever you do something, put all of your effort into it, including rest.
- Take time to get better at tasks by educating yourself and improving your skills.
- Manage your time and energy. Do not waste any of them unnecessarily.

Once you start taking these action steps seriously, you will notice yourself accomplishing a lot more. I will now get into looking towards your future and the life you want to create.

Chapter 3: Visualizing a Better Future

When you learn to get things done and do them well, you will create a better future for yourself. This can become one of your motivations to get moving, as well. In this chapter, I will continue to focus on action steps to get you moving so you can get things done. Once you can visualize your future, you can create it.

How to Visualize Your Future

In this section, I will go over some ways to visualize your future so that you can create an image that inspires you. This is a powerful tool that helps you create the future you want. Will it turn out exactly as you see it? Definitely not. There are too many variables that factor in. However, always keeping that picture in mind means that you will push yourself harder to achieve the success you want. As you see your reality a few years down the line, you will expect more out of yourself. Start by answering the following questions. Remember, these are the answers you hope to give five, 10, 15, or whatever years down the line.

- When someone asks you what you do for work, what do you tell them?
- Describe all of your surroundings in great detail, including your house, the city, neighborhood, and what's nearby. Where do you spend most of your free time?
- What is the atmosphere like at work and in your home, and how do you contribute to it?
- What is your greatest accomplishment? What brings you the most pride?

- Are there any regrets that you have?
- What are the specific steps you took to get where you are?
- What advice would you give to someone else who wants to be where you are?
- What problems arose along the way?

After answering these questions, you will understand where you want to be and have an idea of how to get there.

More Tips for Visualization

Once you begin visualizing your future, then you have it ingrained in your mind. It becomes much harder to let it go. Of course, this does not mean that it's a guarantee. You still must put in the work and make the right moves. For example, if you want to start a business, you can picture the type, how big it will be, where it should be located, how it will look, and whether you plan to have employees or not, among other things. Seeing is believing, though, and the following tips will help you start believing in yourself and your future.

Visualize Your New Life

One way to become excited about your goals is to imagine what your life will be like when you achieve them. For example, if you plan on increasing your salary, imagine that extra money coming in. How much will it be, and what will you be able to do with it? What will you be doing to get that extra money, whether it's through work, investing, or starting a business, etc.? Anything you can imagine about what your life will be like, try to picture it in your mind.

Create a Vision Board

Start collecting images, quotes, articles, and any other visual representations that you feel reflect your future. For instance, you can collect a specific item from a state if you plan on living there someday. This will help you trigger inspiration and hold you accountable for your dreams.

Write Down Your goals

This is a common practice and is touted as being very effective by most productive people. If you are not fond of vision boards, you can write down your goals in lieu of that practice. You may also do it in conjunction with each other for added benefits.

Let Yourself Zone Out

If you find yourself daydreaming at certain times, let it happen. Your mind is trying to tell you something about what you want. Many geniuses in the past, including Einstein, would zone out throughout the day. During these moments, a bolt of inspiration can strike, and great plans can be made. Of course, you cannot daydream all the time, or nothing will get done, which defeats the purpose.

However, when you can, take the time to do it.

Say Your Goals Out Loud

Whatever you have planned, whether short-term or long-term, say it out loud, so the universe knows. This also triggers your brain to understand what you want, so it also starts thinking towards that direction.

Think About What You Want and not What You Don't Want

There is a phenomenon known as the Law of Attraction. According to the rules, what you focus on is what the universe delivers to you, even if you're thinking about it in a negative way. So, even if you're thinking about poverty in terms of not falling into it, you will still attract it because it is in your mind. Therefore, it is better not to even visualize poverty but just think about becoming wealthy.

Life When You Get Things Done

All the information and strategies I have gone over in this book lead up to one thing: Getting things done. That is how you achieve what you want in life. You simply must take action and go for what you want. The action steps in the previous chapters provide a way to make goal-getting easier by providing direction, focus, and motivation. I will end this book by over the many benefits of getting things. Getting things done, or GTD is an actual process and state of mind. When you start incorporating it, you will notice many changes during and after.

A Feeling of Relaxed Control

You will feel in control of your life because you are taking active steps to create it. This may be the number one benefit of getting things done. Performing frequent assessments, processing information, and acting on it can make your mind feel like it's water, where it just flows and makes decisions naturally. It takes time for everyone to get to this state.

Your Thinking Will Be Stimulated

When you get things done, your thinking will be stimulated in advance. You will continuously be thinking about the little and big projects in your life, and they will rarely if ever, slip by you. Procrastination will be an afterthought, and you will always be ahead of the curve.

More Organization and Less Clutter

Getting things done means you will clean off your desk literally and figuratively. You will accomplish your tasks and keep your work area organized too. When you get things done, you will be more versatile, and it will become easier to make and keep commitments. In addition, you will be able to keep others accountable for their commitments.

Less Time for Worry

Thinking is good, but overthinking can be detrimental. It can lead to worry, anxiety, and fear. One of the best ways to avoid this is by acting. Worrying occurs when you have a moment for it. When you act, you are doing and have less time to worry.

The entire point of getting things done is just that, getting things done. This is how you accomplish your goals and start living the life you imagine. There are so many get-rich-quick schemes and people promising others the world if they just do a few simple things. With this book, I wanted to provide many different action steps for you so you can tidy up, clear out unnecessary garbage, both emotional and physical, and start working on your dreams. It may take time, but if you're moving in the right direction, that is what matters most.

PART II

Chapter 1: The Clutter in Your Life

You have probably seen many shows on television about how people hoard several different items, either because they love to shop, or they have collected many articles over time and cannot bear to part with them. It gets to the point where their closets and even their entire homes are filled up completely, and it is nearly impossible to move around. You may know people like this in your own life, or perhaps, you are one of these people. If you are reading this book, then I will assume that the clutter in your space is taking over your life.

Especially in Western society, we have a fascination with material possessions of all types. If we like something, we must have it right away. As a result, we end up purchasing so many different items, and we cannot bear to part with them, even if we don't use them anymore. After several years, our living spaces and office spaces are cluttered. This includes places like the kitchen, living room, and restrooms. So many items get collected that they end up getting stored wherever they can.

You might be wondering what the big deal is. So what if I, or anyone else, collects a lot of items? Well, the stuff is yours, and you have every right to do whatever you want with it. However, what I want to address are the psychological issues that result in clutter building up in your life, as well as the effects the same clutter has on your psyche in the long run.

Why You Have Clutter

There are numerous reasons why you have so much clutter in your life. It is not as simple as forgetting to do your Spring cleaning. Even though this could be a part of it, however, there are deeper issues as well that may reflect certain aspects of your personality. This may be more common than you think because some people are able to artfully hide their clutter behind lock doors, where you will not find it unless you dig deep. You may be hiding your own clutter so that it's not visible to you. However, when you open a certain closet, a few drawers in the house, or walk into your garage or basement, and they are filled with items that you never use, then you may have an issue with clutter.

To be fair, it's almost impossible to have no clutter at all. Having a few extra items on your desk, or a drawer with some junk in the house is not a big deal. However, if it starts to cramp your personal space, then you might have a problem. I will go over some of the main reasons why people have clutter in their homes. See which ones you can relate to.

You Don't Recognize What Clutter Is

Many people allow clutter to build up in their homes because they don't recognize what it is. They have a hard time deciphering between what is valuable and what is just taking up space. Some items were once valuable but haven't been used for a long time. Because it can be hard to recognize what clutter is, people have a hard time letting anything go. They will look at something, suspect that it could come in handy down the line, and then never get rid of it.

You Don't Know How Long You Should Keep Something

This is a huge area of confusion in almost any household. How are you supposed to tell how long to keep something? Many people have no concept of when and where to let things go. I am not just talking about tools or appliances here. This can be related to anything. For example, people still have birthday or holiday cards that are decades old. It is nice to look at these cards and conjure up some nice old memories, but how many reminders of the past do you actually need?

You Don't Know How to Store Things

People often do not know how to store things. It might be because they forget, or they do not know where it should go. Suddenly, you will find something hidden in the weirdest section of your house, or worse, not be able to find it when you need it.

Along the same lines, you have no good organizing routine. Perhaps you are not an organized person, in general. This is not an indictment on you personally. Many individuals lack the ability to organize everything in their lives, and this grows worse with the more items they obtain. You can actually declutter for about

15-20 minutes a day for several days straight, and many of your items will disappear.

You Are Not Using Clutter Busters

Clutter busters are items, such as trays, baskets, jars, hooks, or folders, that can be used to place your materials in specialized locations. Yes, you will still have the items in your home, but at least they won't be in your way all the time. Can you imagine having a toilet brush on your coffee table? I certainly hope not.

Buying Too Many Things, You Don't Need

This is probably the most obvious one. How many of us don't buy things we don't need? From aspirational shopping to impulse buying, our homes are filled with things we bought on a whim. Aspirational shopping comes from our interest in actually doing something, only to realize it's not for us. However, we don't take the time to get rid of the items afterward. For example, we might watch a musician playing the guitar and want to be like him. So, we buy a guitar, end up hating it, or get to busy to practice, and then put it in a closet somewhere.

If you genuinely have an interest in learning something, I think it's great. But at least stick to it for a little while to give it a chance. If you end up not liking it, then sell the items or donate them to someone who will use them.

In this last instance, you may know you are a clutter bug, and may not want to be one, but you can't seem to let things go. You have a weird attachment to them and might not know why. This will require a deeper understanding of who you are and why particular items are hard to let go, even if you never use them.

Assess your own situation and determine which of these reasons are causing you to hold onto clutter. It might be a combination of things, which is fine. The important thing is to recognize why the spaces in your life seem so busy when they do not have to be.

Endowment Effect

There is a phenomenon known as the endowment effect, which can also explain why people have a hard time getting rid of things. This is a type of bias that occurs when people overvalue something simply because they own it. It might have been given to them, or they bought it years ago, but would never consider getting it now. However, since they own it, they place a greater worth on it.

This psychological bias has resulted in many people not being able to part with something. They are not even willing to sell it at a fair price, because they feel no one will pay the real value of it. The ironic part is the person with the attachment would never consider buying the article for nearly the same price they are trying to sell it for. For example, if they have a special coffee mug, they will put it on the market for $10, but if they saw the mug in a store, they will not even consider purchasing it. It seems that ownership gives people a certain sense of power, and they hate giving it up.

There is also a concept in psychology known as loss aversion. This is where people feel the pain of losing something at a higher intensity than the joy of gaining something of equal value. For example, if a person loses five dollars, but then finds five dollars somewhere else, the original pain of losing money will still affect them more than the joy of finding money. This can be another reason the endowment effect is so powerful. If a person owns an item, getting rid of it in exchange for the actual value will not be acceptable to them. Therefore, individuals who are impacted by this mindset will overly price something to compensate for their feelings of loss.

The endowment effect is an interesting bias that is still being studied today. It is not completely understood why this mindset affects people. But it definitely does.

The Consequences of Too Much Clutter

While you may think that too much clutter just means you will have a hard time moving around stuff, the consequences actually go much deeper than that. There are numerous negative results that happen due to excess clutter, and some of them might surprise you. After this, you will probably be more motivated to clean up a little bit.

Your Stress Levels Increase

People who live in cluttered environments have higher levels of stress and fatigue. Even increased amounts of the stress hormone, cortisol, was found in their blood. Because individuals stayed in these environments, their cortisol levels never dropped throughout the day, causing chronic stress, more chronic disease risks, and even greater mortality risk.

Your Diet Is Impacted in A Negative Way

Psychological studies have also shown that people who live in more orderly environments tend to choose healthier snack options that those in cluttered areas. Since stress leads to unhealthy snacking, being around too much clutter will lead to poor dietary habits. People also tend to overeat with too much stress.

You Can Develop More Respiratory Issues

Homes that are cluttered tend to attract more dust because there are extra physical items it can settle on top of. Extra dust in the air can eventually lead to respiratory issues in the long run, and can also exacerbate active problems, like asthma or COPD.

The more items you have inside your home, the more dust is generated. This will also attract dust mites. Furthermore, if your clutter gets way too excessive, then several areas of your home will become exceedingly difficult to reach and clean. As a result, more dust will build up. Of course, respiratory issues can lead to even more health consequences.

Your Safety Is Threatened

Too much clutter can lead to an unsafe environment where people can trip and fall easily. You also have more items to bump into when you can't see. In addition, it can be difficult to move around, and essential exits might be blocked. This causes a huge risk if you ever have to evacuate your home urgently. A fire can also spread much more quickly if you have a lot of combustible items lying around.

Your Love Life Is Jeopardized

Clutter can negatively affect marriages, too, as people who have difficulty parting with things may build resentment in their spouse. The clutter does not just impact you, but everyone else in your home too. If the person you love is bothered by the clutter and you're not, then your marriage can definitely suffer.

If you are not married and just dating, imagine what your date would think if she saw your home, and it is completely disorganized. If they don't run for the hills right away, they might do so as soon as the date is over.

Your Kids Will Be Upset

Yes, your kids, who you constantly tell to clean their room, will be upset with excess clutter. Studies have found that kids who live in a cluttered environment tend to have more distress, which will affect other areas of their lives.

You Will Become Isolated

A large number of adults say they won't invite anyone over to their house if they feel it is too messy. If you have a lot of clutter and you feel this way, then you likely have not had many guests in your house recently. This can cause you to become isolated from the world, especially if you are a homebody. If you like to spend all of your time outside of your home, then I guess this one won't be too relevant for you.

A person who lives in clutter rarely confines these tendencies to their home life. They will carry them everywhere, including their work environment, as you will see with some of the following examples.

You Will Miss Out On Getting Promoted

Untidiness at work, including a messy desk, a chaotic briefcase, or an unorganized filing system, can have negative impacts on your job performance. You will likely spend too much time looking for things and not enough time actually doing any work. Your boss will notice your clutter as well, and this can put you in a bad light when it's time to hand out promotions. According to a study on the career website, CareerBuilder, roughly 28% of employers are less likely to promote someone who keeps their workspace messy. They feel that disorganization leads to poor job performance, and they are right to think this way.

You Are More Likely to Miss Work

The National Institute of Mental Health studies have found that individuals in a cluttered environment are more likely to miss work. They estimated an average of seven missed days per month, which is an excessive number.

Your Productivity Decreases

While you are in a cluttered environment, your ability to focus is severely impeded. If you have many different items within your visual field simultaneously, they all compete for your brain's attention. You cannot give it equally to all of them, so you focus more on things that you are interested in. More often than not, that usually not your work projects. If you have papers, pens, food, and various other things on your desk, you will have a hard time getting any work done at all, and your productivity will be greatly affected. Once again, the bosses will take notice, and you won't be in very high standing when they hand out raises or promotions. In fact, they may not keep you at all if you're not performing as you should.

See how many negative results can happen to your career by keeping your workspace too cluttered? It will behoove you and your career aspirations to change this quickly.

You Will Develop Poor Spending Habits

When you live in a cluttered environment, it can become difficult to find things. As a result, you will buy another item of the same kind, not realizing it was hiding under all of your rubbish.

You Can Go into Debt

This last one may not be relevant anymore due to the ability to make online payments, but those of you who rely on paper bills as a reminder to pay them will suffer greatly. Bills become lost and forgotten, resulting in extra fees. If these are really important bills like credit cards or house payments, then additional problems will occur with the banks and financial institutions. Even your credit score will start to decline.

As you can see, the various negative effects of too much clutter can impact every area of your life. It can significantly decrease your physical and mental health and create many psychological issues for you. With the impact on career and relationships too, you will fall further down into the abyss.

Think about your own life and determine how much of an effect clutter has on your mindset. I am willing to bet that you feel much better sitting in a particular area after you have cleaned it up a little bit. Now that we have established some reasons why people collect clutter and the negative consequences associated with it, I will go over some action steps to get rid of clutter in your life.

Clutter is Not Just Physical

I have spoken a lot about the physical clutter around your home or office. All of this is very distracting and can cause you to lose focus. Too many stimuli will compete for your focus, and you will not be able to give any of them your full attention. Important issues will go right over your head.

Physical clutter is bad, but it is not the only kind you have to contend with. Clutter also includes technology, which is a growing problem in this day and age. We get emails all the time from many different sources. Sometimes we don't even know who the email is from, and just ignore it. However, we often don't erase the email or unsubscribe from the individual, which results in even more unnecessary items in our inbox. Junk email is literally regular junk mail on steroids. When we get so many different ones from various sources, it clutters our files, and we become extremely overwhelmed, just like with physical clutter. As a result, a lot of important information falls through the cracks.

With so much information coming in, it becomes very distracting, and our ability to focus and remain productive decreases. Once we become overwhelmed, we no longer answer emails; we simply scroll through them and hope we did not miss anything important. Suddenly, an important email from our boss comes through, and we never catch it. As a result, critical information was missed, which can jeopardize your company and even your job.

Digital clutter is not exclusive to too many emails. Having an excessive number of programs or apps on your computer, carrying around multiple devices, managing multiple social media accounts, and storing a lot of photos can also be overwhelming in the same manner. In many cases, once a person's data gets used up, they just buy more space, rather than clearing out what they have. It's usually quicker and easier that way. It may not seem like a big deal in the present moment, but after a few months or years, you will realize just how much your productivity and focus has decreased. Increasing productivity and getting things done will be a major topic of this book.

Chapter 2: Breaking Your Relationship With "Stuff"

Now that we have established the psychological reasons people hold onto things, it is to incorporate strategies that will help you get rid of excess clutter. While decluttering can be very difficult at first, it can also be very freeing and have a positive impact on your life in every way. In this chapter, I will go over various different techniques for you to start reducing your personal items or reorganizing them in a proper fashion. Either way, your home, and workspace will become more appealing and habitable.

Getting Over the Endowment Effect

Since the Endowment effect has such a great impact on your ability to get rid of things, I will go over some tips to help you overcome it. Once you go through these steps, you will realize how little value the items in your life actually have and how ridiculous it was to hold onto them for so long when you weren't using them.

The following are a few simple ways to get over the endowment effect:

- Well, now that you know what the endowment effect is, you can become aware that it is personally affecting your life. If you are having difficulty

letting go of something you don't need, tell yourself it's the endowment effect and break the curse.
- Using your imagination can help here too. If you are having a hard time getting rid of something, imagine that you do not own it anymore. This can help weaken the emotional ties you have to it.
- Take the items you no longer use and put them in a sealed box. Now, put them somewhere like an attic or basement. Give yourself a timeline, like three months or six months, and if you do not open that box, then give it away without unsealing it.
- Write down your "why." Why is it important for you to declutter, and what value will it bring to your life?

These tips will help you overcome the power that the endowment effect holds on you, and it should become a little easier to declutter your life after this.

More Decluttering Tips

In this section, I will go over some more decluttering tips to help you reorganize your life. You can use one, or all of these, to start getting rid of unnecessary items. Through some of these steps, you can also determine which items you still need and the ones you can get rid of without a thought.

- Make the process less overwhelming if you are new. Start with five minutes a day and use this time to declutter what you can. From here, raise the time at your comfort level.

- Give one item away each day. By the end of week one, you will have given away seven items. By the end of the year, you will have given away 365. You will definitely see your belongings disappearing quickly. If you want to make the process faster, you can certainly increase the amount you give away.

- Get a large trash bag and fill it up with as many items as you can. After filling it up, tie the bag and donate to Goodwill or another donation service before you change your mind.

- Take all of your clothes and hang them facing backward. Whenever you wear an item, hang them back up facing forward. After several months, the clothes that are still facing backward should be donated.

- Use the 12-12-12 rule for getting rid of items. Take out 12 things that you plan on donating, 12 things that you plan to throw away, and 12 things that you will keep for now. This will lessen the impact of getting rid of things because you can see what you're still keeping.

- Go into your home with a first-time visitor mindset. Look around the house and determine how you would clean and reorganize the place, including what items you would get rid of. This is a mind trick you can use to detach yourself from the things inside.

- Choose a small area of your home and take before and after pictures. For example, take a small section on your kitchen counter that has clutter, snap a quick photo, and then clean off the area. Take another photo right after that. Having this visual will help you keep that area clear. Start doing this with other areas of your home too.

Decide whichever tip works best for you and then go from there. If there are others that you come up with, that is fine too. The goal is to declutter in whatever way necessary, so get creative in your approach.

Stop Buying Stuff You Don't Need

If you are decluttering the stuff out of your personal space, but also buying things you don't need at the same time, then it defeats the purpose. You are just replacing one set of items for another. As a result, decluttering will mean nothing as your environment will just become busy again. The goal of decluttering is to keep your space from becoming overfilled. This requires a combination of getting rid of stuff and not buying new stuff. The following are some effective ways to stop buying unnecessary items.

Keep Away from Temptations

If you have a tendency to splurge on things you don't need, then don't tempt yourself by window shopping or going into a store to look around. You might also want to stop getting shopping magazines and cancel online subscriptions to stores. You may not be thinking about buying an item until you see it, and then suddenly, it is in your room just sitting there.

If you must go to the store, make a list and stay laser-focused on it. If you know where the items are, then only go to those sections of the store. You can also shop online and have the items delivered, so you don't actually go out.

Avoid Retail Seduction

Retail stores are masterful at seduction, from hiring the best salespeople, to proper lighting, placement, and layout. All of this is done to draw in their customers, and many people fall for it. This is why someone ends up spending 20 dollars on a coaster set when a five-dollar one would have worked.

Avoid retail seduction by being aware of it. When you see an enticing item, mentally isolate it from its environment and see if the appeal is still there. Also, imagine it being placed in a bin at the thrift store and see if you still want to buy it.

Take Inventory

Oftentimes, we buy things because we don't have enough. However, if you take regular inventory of everything in your home, including inside the drawers, you will find more than you realized. The desire to buy more will go down. Even after you declutter, you will still have many items.

Practice Gratitude

Be mindful of the things you have in your life, both tangible and intangible, and show gratitude for them. Again, you will realize your life is more fulfilling than it appeared beforehand.

These are just a few tips to keep you from going on a shopping splurge and refilling your house with items that are useless. Once you see the powerful effects that decluttering will have on you, it will be lifechanging in so many ways. This is why so many people who became minimalists are much happier now.

Calculate Cost Vs. Labor

The trick here is to figure out how much something costs, and then determine how many hours you would have to work to make up that money. This can really be eye-opening for you. Determine if the labor hours are worth the item you want to purchase.

Keep Your Big Picture in Front of You

When you are spending money day-to-day, it can be easy to lose track of things. You may not realize how much one day of spending can take you away from your ultimate goals. This is why it's important to keep the big picture at the forefront of your mind. Use whatever reminders you need to accomplish this.

A lot of the techniques I have gone over about tricking your mind or shifting the mindset away from what you are used to. Incorporating all of these strategies into your life on a regular basis will give you the best results.

The Benefits Of Decluttering

The benefits of decluttering are another thing you can keep in mind to help you stay focused on eliminating excessive items from your life. The process really is freeing once you give it a chance. The following are a summary of some of the benefits of decluttering. I will get into many more over the next few sections.

- Reduced stress and anxiety related to all of the clutter.
- Reduced number of allergens, like dust, pet hair, and pollen that can accumulate on surfaces.
- A cleaner and more sanitary environment.
- Save extra money and even make money by selling things.
- Extra space in your home for fun activities.
- Less shame in inviting guests.
- Your home will be safer to move around in. There will be fewer things to run into.
- Family or others who are living with you will appreciate it.
- You will realize how many things you can actually do without.

Decluttering Equals Increased Focus and Productivity

Imagine a housecat for a moment. They easily become distracted by shiny lights, new toys, or any hanging objects. If you put something in front of a cat's face, they will be mesmerized by it. If you place multiple items in front of them, they will not be able to figure out which one to focus on. Our minds can become the same way if we let them.

Lucky for us, our brains have a natural filtering mechanism that allows it to not be distracted by every little thing around is. So, when you are performing a task, you may not notice the slight wind outside, the cars driving by on the front seat, or every single person that walks by. Our brains do a great job of shutting out what we don't need to see, hear, or feel every moment.

The problem here is, it takes a lot of energy to filter things out, and this energy is finite. This means that the more things around us that have the potential to catch our attention, the more energy the brain uses, and the more quickly it will dissipate. Therefore, the more clutter you have, the quicker your brain will lose its ability to focus, and you will become distracted more easily.

It is simple to see, then, that decluttering will increase your focus because you have fewer things that will drain the energy required to keep it. Try something as soon as you can. While you are sitting at your table, remove a few items from it and see how many less distractions you have. Remove any objects that are unnecessary to the task at hand. Many people will keep snacks at their desks. Avoid doing this because then you will just be snacking constantly, instead of working. When you're hungry, actually get up, and make yourself something. Put in the work.

Notice how much clearer your mind feels after doing this. When our surroundings become too busy, so does our mind. While some people believe that a busy mind creates productivity, it is quite the opposite. A clear mind with focus is what allows true productivity, so if you want to get things done, clear up your environment, and clear up your brain.

Decluttering and Improved Health

Decluttering will improve many aspects of your health. Notice some of the healthiest people around you, and you will see that their living or workspaces are immaculate compared to others. I will go over a few ways that decluttering will have positive health consequences.

Improved Healthy Habits

When you declutter your home, you will develop healthy habits. The main reason for this is that certain items will be easier to get to and will more likely get used. For example, if you open your closet and quickly find the vacuum or broom, you are more likely to use them. If your vacuum is behind a wall of various items, you will not want to put in the effort to get it. This goes for cooking, as well. If your kitchen is filled up with supplies, like extra appliances, cookware, dirty dishes, and various articles that don't need to be there, you are less likely to cook meals at home. There is a greater chance that you'll just cook a microwave dish or buy fast food.

Better Self-Care

When living in a clean and sanitary environment, you will have better self-care overall. It will be easier and more appealing to exercise in an open space. Also, your sleeping habits will improve because it is easier to be restful in less busy surroundings. Finally, people who declutter slowly develop the habit of remaining clean, which improves hygienic practices.

Losing Weight

This may seem like an odd connection, but it's true. People are much more likely to be overweight if they live in a cluttered environment. A study done by the University of Florida estimates about a 77 percent higher chance of being overweight or obese. This is related to the busy lifestyles that people have, which is common with people who do not declutter. When you learn to declutter, you also learn to slow down. You also become much more organized. This gives you more time to eat properly and exercise.

Easier to Relax

Too much clutter in your home can impact your ability to relax and enjoy yourself. The immense amount of distractions will ever allow your mind to stop getting distracted. It will be hard to immerse yourself in a relaxing activity, like reading, watching a movie, or taking a bath. You will just feel cramped, and trying to calm your nerves will be an uphill batter you cannot win.

All of these benefits will work in conjunction to improve your physical and mental health.

Having More Space

It is easy to see that decluttering opens up space around you. Not only will you have a greater physical area to work in, but a larger mental space to think. You will become more creative because it will be easier for you to open up your mind. This is where some of your best ideas will come into play.

Having an open space can increase your confidence and self-efficacy. A lot of this has to deal with the decluttering process. As you remove items from your life or reorganize them, you will have to make some important decisions. Getting rid of stuff is not easy, and you will have to think quite a bit. This will improve your capability to come up with solutions, which will definitely make you more confident in yourself. This will also give you more energy because you put yourself in the mode of getting things done. This relates back to productivity.

Having more open space reduces family and relationship tension. An excessive mess can lead to major arguments. Disagreements may arise over who causes the clutters, and therefore, who should get rid of it. Parents will often become frustrated with their children because it will take forever to find something. Do not underestimate how beneficial having more open space can be for your personal relationships.

Think back to when you moved into your home or office. This was prior to moving in any furniture or personal items. Even if it's a small space, it certainly looked much bigger than it appeared before adding extra items. Now, imagine how much bigger your space will become from just removing half of your stuff out. You will truly appreciate the extra space when you have it.

6-Week Decluttering Challenge

You can certainly take as long as you need to declutter your home, office, car, or other space that you occupy regularly, but using a challenge can light a fire under and hold you accountable for making some real changes. You can also bring in the help of a friend to help hold you accountable. Let them know what you plan to accomplish each week, and then bring them in at the end of every week to assess your progress. Take before and after photos, too, so you can have your own visuals.

It is a simple process. Starting from the beginning, pick a certain part of your home that you will focus on each week. For example, week one will be dedicated to the kitchen and dining room. Then, the second week will be dedicated to the living room. The third week will be dedicated to one or two bedrooms, depending on the amount of clutter. In the fourth week, the focus will be on the garage. In the fifth week, you can start on the basement. Finally, the sixth week can be used for any leftover closets or the laundry room. This is just an example, and you can make up your own plan based on your particular spaces. You can break down each week into smaller goals, as well.

Here is a visual:

- Week 1: Kitchen and dining room
    - Declutter the countertops-Day 1
    - Declutter the fridge-Day 2
    - Declutter the cabinets-Day 3
    - Declutter the pantry-Day 4
    - Declutter the stove and oven-Day 5
    - Declutter the dining room table-Day 6
    - Declutter any other tables or cabinets in the dining room-Day 7

It may be best to start in the kitchen because it is a high traffic area in the house. From here, you can cover the other areas of your home and break it down day by day. It is really that simple. You just have to maintain discipline. Feel free to incorporate any of the strategies for decluttering I went over earlier.

After doing the six-week challenge, give yourself a pat on the back for your accomplishment. You can even reward yourself. In fact, you can also give yourself small rewards at the end of each week, granted that you accomplished what you needed to. If you stick to the challenge, you will not believe how much more space you will have. Your home may even look bigger than before.

Now that we have established the benefits of decluttering and how you can get this done in your life, the rest of the book will cover how to move forward and start getting things done in your life.

PART III

Chapter 1: Is This for You?

Before we start this adventure, we have to ask, who is this intended for? The short answer is that it is for everyone who wants to make a positive change in their lives. The key word there is "want". This is ultimately a choice. You must establish your own journey as the techniques exemplified in this book are just practices. There is no set number of meditation sessions that will unlock mindfulness. The practice of these techniques only increases the chances of your own self-discovery. Your willingness to find that goal is the only way these practices will be effective.

This may seem confusing or even overwhelming, but it should be celebrated! You have made a choice to better your life. You possess the bravery to examine yourself in your own state. You are already stronger for it. There is value in yourself and your life and you have already made the decision to discover yourself at your most honest, happiest state and to continue to not only endure but thrive in a world made by your own choices. The biggest step is the first one, and that step is already behind you. It is time to breathe a sigh of relief, to feel accomplished. The worst part of your journey is behind you.

Now that you have made the first step, where do you go? Obviously, the answer is your own choice. The practices in this book are merely there to help you along the way. This may or may not be a path that you have previously gone down, so use these techniques to guide you in your own journey. Look at this book as a toolkit. There is nothing in these pages that will assume a role of authority over you. That is the beauty of free will! You are free to explore at your own pace in your own order.

"Often, it's not about becoming a new person, but becoming the person you were meant to be, and already are, but don't know how to be."

— Heath L. Buckmaster, Box of Hair: A Fairy Tale

You have already made the most important step, and that step is the one that separates you from your furthest setbacks. There is already so much distance between where you were and where you are now. It is now possible to look back and accept yourself. Standing where you are now, it is possible to see your own worth. You are not your setbacks, and you are not your failures. In fact, you might be the most interesting person you know!

Chapter 2: Your Toolbox, DBT

The goal of Dialectical Behavior Therapy (DBT) is to separate you from behaviors that are harmful to yourself and others and replace them with meaningful habits. Now that you have taken your first step and have separated yourself from your setbacks, you can go even further and discover what it is that makes you truly happy on your own. Finding that you do not live to continue harmful behaviors but discovering and tailoring habits that will enhance the life that you are choosing to live will fill you with serenity and self-love, and it will be all the more meaningful because they will be your own interests and not the consequences of your setbacks. Honestly, how exciting is it to really discover the real you? Someone that you may have never met or may not have seen in a long time and neither has anyone else, a brand-new person who has been there all along.

The defined objectives of DBT is obviously a little more clinical. It includes Mindfulness, Distress Tolerance, Interpersonal Effectiveness, and Emotion Regulation. How does this relate to you, though? How do these skills fit into your new and exciting life? Remember that the goal of this kind of therapy is not to overtake your life, but to be there alongside it to help you discover what it is that makes you the real you.

Mindfulness is not a skill set, more so a state of being. Mindfulness is being aware of the present, in the present, and not to be overwhelmed by what is going on around you. It is an awesome way to be and reinforces who you are because only you have a mind like yours. Whenever you are using your senses to become directly aware of your present state of being, you are being mindful. Mindfulness is also exercised like a muscle. It is something that we all possess, but few regularly practice. Although that statement may not be true for long. There is a growing interest in meditation and a growing awareness of the importance of remaining mindful in every aspect of life from personal to even business. If you were to practice it, you will discover that the feeling of mindfulness becomes stronger the more you exercise that mental muscle. Focus and personal honesty will become stronger as you develop along this path. It is an exciting tool of self-discovery and one that will be explored upon later in this book.

Distress Tolerance is a measurement. It is your ability to accept distress that cannot be changed. Emotional pain is measured on a different scale altogether from physical pain, but it can be just as, or even more, damaging. The real skill here is learning how to find your own way around the distress and accept what you are unable to change. Practicing mindfulness will help you to separate yourself from distress factors but coming to terms with the reality of these stressful situations will no longer be a roadblock, but a defining challenge that will make you stronger and give you skills for future distress management.

"Grant me the serenity, to accept the things I cannot change; courage to change the things I can; and wisdom to know the difference."

Learning the difference between what you can and cannot control is paramount. Once you have accepted the reality of a stressful situation that you cannot control, you cease to try to change it but begin to find a path to live around or through it. Sometimes, the energy spent trying to change an unchangeable situation is more stressful than the original event! You owe it to yourself to not harm yourself. There are even times when the situation only seems to be so stressful because you have spent all of your energy and effort trying to change it instead of taking a step back and accepting it for what it is. You could even come to realize that the situation is more benign than how you have built it up to be inside your head. Sometimes, you can even find a way to turn it into a positive situation! You will never be able to do any of that if you are too busy stressing about the original situation, though.

Interpersonal Effectiveness will help you to build and maintain important relationships, including the one you have with yourself, as well as help you to define priorities and to arrange them in a sensible manner to live your new life the most effective. The clinical method is through the acronym DEAR MAN:

- **D**escribe the current situations
- **E**xpress your feelings and opinions
- **A**ssert yourself by asking for what you want, or by saying no
- **R**eward the person – let them know what they will get out of it
- **M**indful of objectives without distractions (attack the problem, not the person)
- **A**ppear effective and competent
- **N**egotiate alternative solutions

These are effective and healthy steps for conflict resolution and a great tool to have in mind to keep your communication on track and working towards an agreeable solution.

Respect is a trait valued by everybody in one way or another. Respect is earned and kept and can encourage stronger relationships with the important people in your life. Speaking in a respectful tone will lead you to your interpersonal goals in a way than getting agitated towards that person, situation, or even yourself. Self-respect is the true basis of interpersonal respect. Have you ever heard that you must learn to love yourself before you can love another? This is because you define for yourself, and exemplify to others, what respect means to you. How you treat yourself will set the standard for how others will feel that they can treat you. A person who dresses nice and speaks warmly with peers will garner more respect than a person who shows little care for how they want to be treated. Self-respect is important, and you deserve it! You are already stronger for having taken this journey and your story is one that no one else has. You are worthwhile, interesting, and unique. Taking good care of yourself will tell others that you are a person who warrants respect. Another acronym that is helpful about self-respect is FAST.

- **F**air to myself and others
- No **A**pologies for being alive
- **S**tick to values (do not do anything you will regret later)
- **T**ruthful without excuses or exaggeration

You have heard the Golden Rule; treat others as you would like to be treated yourself. Well, that rule works the other way as well! Treat yourself as you would treat others. You deserve the same respect that you would show to others, so do not count yourself out or make sacrifices that make you feel uncomfortable. Be fair to yourself!

If you find that you apologize unnecessarily, stop it! Sometimes, people will tell you that you apologize too much, which only make you feel uncomfortable. You do not have to apologize for anything that you are not truly sorry for. You occupy the same space as your peers and you deserve the same level of respect.

What are your values? Do you know? In your current stage of rebuilding and discovery, your values may change, or you may discover that you have been violating your own values for a long time. With a renewed respect for yourself and a bright new path ahead of you, you are most likely to find out what is truly important to you. Find your core values and remember that you deserve respect. You do not have to apologize for your values and you do not have to compromise your values. Make your identity known and remember that you are valid.

Once you know who you are, what you value, and the fact that you deserve and possess self-respect, honesty becomes easy. You do not have to fabricate yourself to fit in or hide any unsavory traits that you may think that you possess. Your peers will respect an honest you. Honesty to yourself and others is the pinnacle of freedom. You are who you are and who you are is a strong, healthy, and an interesting person! Half-truths and flat out lies do little more than create stress for everyone involved, including yourself. A person with self-respect does not need to create an identity that they do not own. Breathe and relax because you are you!

Chapter 3: Finding Yourself through Mindfulness

Discovering yourself is exciting! It's a journey that is enviable. We have already defined mindfulness, so the next step is to discover how it is practiced and define what your individual goals are. It is important to remember to constantly ask yourself what you want to find in this book. Your individual goals are the goals of this text. What practitioners of mindfulness usually find is greater fulfillment, a deeper understanding of their selves, positive behavioral changes, and more importantly, less suffering.

As you continue down this path, it is important to remember what your truest intentions are because doubts will surface. Mindfulness will need to be practiced and exercised like a muscle. Minds are messy, prone to wandering, prone to doubt, and everyone examines themselves much harsher than their peers would. In the last chapter, you discovered what your values are and who you are as a person. You discovered that self-respect is worth having. Now, it is time to reinforce what you know about yourself and what you want to explore.

Before we get to the actual practices, it is important to note that the path to mindfulness is not linear. It is a little different for everyone and the only outside guide is a collection of experiences from others. The true guide is yourself. Do not fret. Do not succumb to doubt because you may or may not discover a path differently or find a truth not listed in this book. No one can know you as well as you can. Instead of reveling in the doubt or confusion, be excited! You are the first to discover your exact path and you are the first to find your own unique solutions to your setbacks.

At the same time, you may discover that these goals are even connected! As you discover greater fulfillment, you may connect it to lesser suffering, and from there, you may find that you exhibit better behavior and more success in your relationships. Understand that practicing separateness from your suffering could lead to accepting validation from your own positive thoughts and energy.

The most obvious exercise for practicing mindfulness is meditation. It is important to note that meditation is not passive. It is not simply sitting and relaxing with your eyes closed. It is an active exploration of your mind while providing yourself with the least resistance to your own self-discovery. You may not just drop right into it during your first session. An unpracticed mind has never explored in that way. You may not know how to look inward as your senses and instincts are conditioned to look outward for stimulation.

First, you must separate yourself from your reactions. You must understand what your automatic reactions to a stimulus such as stress and joy are and be aware of yourself at the moment that you act automatically. You are not your feelings. You are not your reactions. Imagine you are on the side of a road watching traffic pass back and forth. Every car is a stimulus, feeling, or reaction. You are separate from them and you must merely make a mental note of it, and then let it pass. Be aware of their existence and acknowledge them, but do not react to them. Eventually, your mind will become more still.

Another example is to imagine your mind like a still pool of water. Every thought and stimulus is a pebble dropped in that pool. Those pebbles create concentric ripples that expand outward, and then even out. If you reach into the water to grab that pebble, you will only create a splash and larger ripples. Eventually, the pebbles will slow, and your quietest realizations and truths will surface. Do not fear! This is your truest self. This is exciting and another great achievement along with your journey to a more peaceful and successful you. After those truths have passed without judgment, your pool of water will fall even more still. You will experience true serenity and discover the most honest definition of a quiet mind. This is peace.

To practice meditation, you must first dedicate time and space to your session. You do not need a special pillow or certain music or any equipment whatsoever, just time and space to practice. Sit in a comfortable position that you will not stress to maintain and close your eyes. Next, just acknowledge the moment as it is. Observe it without judgment or interaction. Just simply be in the moment without exerting effort or energy towards it. Pay attention to the sensations of air passing through your nostrils or the presence of sound in your ears. Let the moment pass through you as you sit peacefully in it. The goal is not simply to be calm, it is to be aware of the moment as it is happening right now without interaction or judgment. The next step is not so much a step, but a reassurance. Judgments will rise. It is inevitable, especially when you are first practicing. Remain calm and remain practicing. Do not succumb to doubt or frustration. Simply make a note of it, and let it pass. This is an excellent practice for learning how to move on from frustration or feelings of grudge in your waking life. If your mind wanders too far off of your initial concentration, keep returning to the sensation of your breath. Focus on the gentle sensation of the in and out of your breathing. Simply be in your awareness.

Meditation is a proven method to reduce stress, increase clarity, and can even positively rearrange your brain chemistry! You will notice your brain will have less chatter in your normal life, and you will be less prone to anxiety. It is a great practice for finding a "third way" around a conflict. It can even open up your creativity and lower your heart rate and blood pressure. As I have mentioned before, it has even begun to appear in modern business practices. Some higher up CEOs have adopted this daily practice to increase their creativity and productivity and reduce their stress level in the fast-paced environment that is business. Everyone from athletes to political figures to your average working man benefits from this simple practice.

If you chose to partake in this particular practice, you are unlikely to regret it. The next chapter will focus on advanced meditation techniques for when you discover that you like this new calmer, more focused you!

Chapter 4: Taking Mindfulness to the Next Level with Advanced Meditation Techniques

If you have chosen to give meditation a try, then congratulations! You should feel proud of yourself for having the courage to try something new. You should feel reinforced in your feelings of solidity in your new and healthy life. You have made an actual effort and have taken real-life actions! This is another moment to look at just how far you have come. How has meditation affected your life already? Do you feel a renewed clarity? This chapter will show you advanced techniques that you can practice to further expand your meditation practices.

An easy form of meditation that you can incorporate in your daily life is called a Walking Meditation. Obviously, this can be done simply while walking, or any form of ambulation that you use to get around. It is an action that you do naturally and has been for years. You probably learned how to walk before you learned how to read! This kind of easy, almost automatic and steady movement is a perfect environment to study your meditation practices.

First, you must stand up straight. Keep your back straight as you practice this. It is important to find the posture that is comfortable and promotes easy steps and focus. Next, place your hands together just above your belly button with your thumbs curled in towards your palms. This position promotes a comfortable posture that brings your focus to your center. Your arms are not swaying, and you feel self-contained and comfortable. Now, let your gaze drop slightly. This will also allow you to focus while being aware of where you are walking to. Just like with normal sitting meditation, try not to get lost in outside stimuli, just simply make a note of them and continue on with your focus inwards. Now, you are ready to take your first step. In the last section, I mentioned that breathing could be used to bring your focus back to your center. In this exercise, you will use your steady footfalls to create a rhythmic cadence for you to keep your central focus on. Notice, without interacting, the sensation of the ground on your feet (or whatever mode of transportation that you would use to get around on your own). Notice as the ground rolls from the back to the front of your foot. Notice the gentle bounce of your body as you move along. Now, do the same with the next step and the next. Make sure to walk at a slightly slower pace than usual. It is not necessary to move ridiculously slow, just make sure that it is at a pace where you are able to focus on your gentle and rhythmic movements and still move along at a comfortable speed.

Benefits of this style of meditation are that it allows you to further exercise your focus outside of the room or environment that you have become comfortable meditating in. It allows you to start connecting that focus to your daily life as you practice maintaining that focus during the natural and unpredictable distractions that occur just in a day out. You will also begin to appreciate the seemingly mundane aspects of your day, bringing focus and renewed eyes to aspects of this wonderful life that may have gone unnoticed or underappreciated previously. A cloud moving in front of the sun might bring certain effects to your attention like the changing colors or temperature of this temporary state. You might find a renewed appreciation for the sun and life in general. A gentle breeze might remind you of how temporary forces in your life are. A passing conversation might show you how calm, focused, and centered you are feeling in the moment versus how frantic and anxious the average person is in their daily life. You will discover all of these things while keeping your focus centered. It is important to not react to any of their thoughts, just simply recognize the existence of these thoughts, and let them pass naturally on their own. Bringing your meditation practices from your sterile environment to the waking world is an excellent practice for learning how to maintain and call upon this state of focus when there are events in your life that may be exciting or stressful.

The next technique is quite the opposite. Instead of walking, this technique is most effective while laying down, but it can be done in a sitting position. It is called a Body Scan, and it is used to focus on your physical wellbeing. It gives the sensation of infusing your body with a healing breath.

First, you must sit or lie in a comfortable position. Do not pick a position or surface that will become uncomfortable or distracting during your meditation. Once you are in a good position, place your hands on your stomach in the same manner in which you did during the Walking Meditation, just above your belly button in a comfortable position that brings your focus to the center of your body in a full rest. Once you are in this position, you might find it easier to focus if you close your eyes. Now, take a few deep breaths. Take note of the moment as you are in it, just like you have practiced in the basic meditation technique. Then bring your attention to your body. Notice the sensation and pressure of the floor or chair on your back or legs. Keep taking deep breaths, but this time, notice the invigorating life that fills your body when you inhale deeply and then feel a deeper sense of relaxation on every exhale. Fall deeper and deeper into your focused state with each incremental breath. You may start to notice more minute sensations such as your pulse under your skin, or little hairs standing up on your arm as your body becomes more relaxed and focus.

Now, bring your focus to your stomach area. If your stomach is tense, let it loose. You might even notice that your entire body relaxes as you release the tension in your stomach. Shift your focus from your stomach to your hands just above that area. See if you can allow your hands to soften even more. Feel your body relax even another level. Now, bring your focus to your arms. Let the tension loose in your shoulders. Let the tension loose in your biceps and forearms. After that, it is time to bring your focus to your neck. Let the muscles in your neck relax. It is perfectly acceptable to let your body shift as your muscles become systematically more relaxed. It is almost bound to happen as you are achieving new levels of relaxation. How relaxed you are now will make your initial assessment when you first lied down seem so distant.

After you have relaxed your neck, then it is time to focus on your jaw. Let that tension go. In your waking life, the average person carries extra tension especially in their jaw, shoulders, and fists without even realizing it. You might perceive yourself as relaxed when in actuality; you are much tenser than what is comfortable. This is one of those realizations that you come across through meditation that is an invaluable lesson that you have taught yourself. After you have rolled your relaxing focus over your entire body, take a mental snapshot of your body as a whole. Notice your body in the same way that you notice passing thoughts in the basic meditation technique. You may realize that your body is yours, but it is not you. Your body is a vessel and a tool for who you really are. That separation is important when you practice meditation. It is what allows you to examine thoughts without attachment. Take one more deep breath and allow your eyes to open, feeling a new sense of invigoration and relaxation.

Congratulations! With these three meditation techniques; the basic meditation, the Body Scan, and the Walking Meditation, you are able to perceive and react to thoughts and stimuli within your mind, your body, and your world in a healthy way. There is nothing that you should not be able to process using these techniques. You now have the tools to tackle any hardships along your journey. On top of that, you now have a new perspective that is exciting to explore as you find new hobbies, relationships, and life choices. Now even simple tasks like breathing, walking, or even just existing can be healing and full of positive energy!

The next chapter will focus on processing negative thought patterns in a healthy way. Now that you have this new perspective and new tools, it should be easy to separate yourself from negative thoughts that may surface from your past or present life. Do not fear! You are ready. You are stronger than you have ever been, and you can tackle any setbacks you have experienced, or are currently experiencing. Take a moment to celebrate where you are versus where you have been!

Chapter 5: Using Your New Tools to Process Negative Emotions

Negative emotions will occur. It is the inevitability that comes with the endless possibilities of life. You cannot reasonably expect to live your entire life and never feel sad, hurt, angry, betrayed, embarrassed, or any other emotion that can be perceived as negative. In this chapter, we will review the skills that you have learned to more effectively process your emotions when an inevitably negative emotion occurs. Through Dialectical Behavior Therapy, Emotion Regulation breaks down into three goals.

1. Understand one's emotions
2. Reduce emotional vulnerability
3. Decrease emotional suffering

The first step begins with a simple truth, and that is emotions are not bad. Even negative emotions are not something to just be avoided. It is impossible, and unhealthy to attempt, to avoid every negative emotion that you will come across in your life. Attachment to negative feelings is what causes real suffering. You learned from the last two chapters how to separate yourself from thoughts and emotions. You simply must acknowledge the emotion and/or event, and then let it pass. It is important to acknowledge these emotions, though. Try to define your emotions clearly. Using phrases like "I feel bad" does not give a clear understanding of how you are feeling. Instead of "bad", expand on that. Pinpoint it by saying you feel frustrated, depressed, anxious, or angry. Understanding what and how you are feeling is integral to processing those feelings. It is also important to understand the difference between primary and secondary emotions.

Primary emotions are reactions to an outside stimulus, and secondary emotions are reactions to those primary emotions. For example, if you felt depressed later about being too angry at a friend, then anger would be the primary emotion while depression would be the secondary emotion. The secondary emotion is a judgment of the primary emotion. Learning how to acknowledge emotions without judgment is essential because secondary emotions are destructive. Also, learning how to process negative events without succumbing to negative emotions is very important. Maybe being angry at the friend was not the proper response when you could have used the DEAR MAN acronym in the second chapter of this book to properly resolve that event and those feelings in a way that would solve the issue and be beneficial to both you and your friend. Remember that emotions are not your identity. Emotions are there just to alert you to stimuli that are beneficial or problematic. How you process and express these emotions is entirely up to you.

Reducing emotional vulnerability will increase the stability of your emotions, simply put. In DBT, the methods for reducing emotional vulnerability is through action. It will teach you to create positive habits and experiences to balance out the negative feelings you might be feeling. An easy acronym to remember for this is PLEASE MASTER.

PL – represents taking care of your physical body and reducing or treating illness
E – eat a balanced diet
A – is for avoiding alcohol and drugs, which can only heighten or fabricate negative feelings
S – Sleep. It is important to get regular sleep
E – The last E is for exercise. Much like meditation, it will increase in benefits the more you practice.
MASTER – This one is the fun one. Master positive activities to increase your sense of well-being and accomplishment.

Your health affects your emotional state. This ties into the self-respect section that we talked about in the second chapter. You will feel much better physically and emotionally if you raise your standards of how you treat yourself. Getting regular sleep, exercise, and only treating your body and yourself to healthy food and activities will do absolute wonders for your confidence. This also includes avoiding alcohol and drugs. It is too easy to mask feelings with these substances, and as we have learned, that is not a healthy way to process those emotions. Avoiding emotions, especially with mind-altering substances, does not make those emotions go away. It is not a permanent solution, it only encourages you to chase that perceived temporary safety from those emotions while your body is developing an addiction to the actual substance. It is a trap and can only work to undo all of the work that you have already accomplished. Treat yourself better than that because not only do you have self-respect, but you deserve it.

Now, I am going to circle back to the PL portion of the PLEASE MASTER acronym. After you understand the steps necessary for taking care of your body, you will understand that it is important to monitor your body as a whole. This includes taking care of illnesses when they arrive. Illness is another inevitability of life. Much like emotions, it is important to process them in a healthy manner to avoid further damage. You deserve to live in a healthy body and you owe it to yourself to take care of yourself. Living in a healthy body will give you peace of mind. Knowing that at the end of the day, you are physically feeling healthy will put other situations in perspective and it will be one more positive that you can weigh against negative emotions when they occur. Along with exercise and meditation, you can choose to MASTER other positive activities in your life. Developing or rediscovering a hobby is exciting and can give new meaning and a new sense of accomplishment in your life!

After you have learned these skills, you are ready to learn how to decrease emotional suffering. In DBT, it is comprised of only two skills: Letting go and taking opposite action.

Letting go refers to what we have already learned, by using our mindfulness to process emotions in a healthy way by letting them pass without developing secondary emotions to attach to the primary emotions. Taking opposite action means engaging in actions that are in direct contrast to the negative feelings that you are experiencing. For example, instead of crying when a feeling of depression is acknowledged, try to stand straight, speak confidently, and react to the stimulus or event in a healthy way. This is not to ignore that emotion. It is an exercise to lessen the length and severity of the emotion. It is important to acknowledge emotions, but that does not mean that you have to be subordinate to them. You do not need to let emotions control how you think and act. It can also give you a new perspective on a situation that you may have reacted automatically too.

With these skills, coupled with the skills you have learned in the previous few chapters, you can process emotions internally in your mind, body, and everyday life and also express those emotions after you have processed them. Even more to add to that, you have developed a renewed sense of self-respect through self-care and new or rediscovered hobbies. You are now taking steps to replace negative habits and feelings with positive feelings and activities you enjoy and that are uniquely representative of you! You may start to feel that you are meeting the real you, a more positive and honest version of yourself, doing things that you enjoy.

Chapter 6: Defining Your Goals, Your Values, and Yourself

Now, instead of learning something new, it is time to reassess yourself after what you have already learned. Do you remember those goals and values that you defined for yourself at the beginning of this book? Well much like how we discovered new levels of relaxation during the Body Scan meditation, it is time to discover new levels of yourself. Maybe after you have practiced meditation and studied the different goals of DBT, your renewed sense of self and awareness can further sharpen your goals and expectations from your new life. It is even possible that you have already achieved and mastered some of your goals. If you have, then congratulations! It is time to reassess what is important to you and what you can get out of this book. If you have not achieved any of your goals yet, then do not worry! Hopefully, you have set expectations at a reasonable level and you are mindful of what you are able to achieve within yourself. It is good to have both long-term and short-term goals. It is important, even, to balance both so you are able to celebrate achievements along the path to a life-affirming goal that you may not have been able to achieve without taking that all important first step along this journey.

Each new skill you learn is a skill you would not have had if you would have maintained your negative feelings and habits. There are questions for you now that only you can answer. How is it that you feel? How do you feel in a general sense of wellbeing? How far along do you think you have traveled? You are most likely aware of your progress and it is good to celebrate along the way. These steps you are taking are not steps that any one person could take for you, no matter how influential or qualified. Just like how meditation and mindfulness is a study of you, the steps you have taken are entirely unique to you.

Having said all of that, it is important to allow positive feelings to be acknowledged and witnessed. Many have a hard time accepting themselves in their own achievements. Judgments upon oneself can absolutely be the harshest. It is easy for faults and negative feelings to seem large and overwhelming when you are standing so near to them. These negative feelings cause you to stress and can be impossible to simply ignore. This is why we learn to process those feelings and resolve them instead of trying in vain to ignore them. An unresolved negative feeling can trigger a survival response, which is why it is impossible to ignore said feelings. In this way, unresolved negative feelings make it near impossible to accept positive feelings about yourself.

Your body does not feel the need to react to positive feelings because it feels that the situation is resolved because it ended on a satisfying conclusion. Your body will tell you that your time and effort need to be spent resolving those negative feelings because they are triggering a survival response in you. Now that you have learned how to bring negative feelings to a positive and productive conclusion, it is now possible to accept your positive traits and individuality. It is even possible to meet yourself without those impossible stresses in your life. How exciting and life-affirming is that! How much better off are you now in relation to how you were before you took this journey?

Now, that you know your goals, and you know yourself, what are your values in your new life now? What have you learned that you could possibly maintain, or even teach others? Maybe you recognize the work that you have put in and are starting to recognize the results of hard work. Maybe you value patience and understanding because practicing meditation has taught you how to discover feelings that were always there, just buried. All this book can do is speculate and give examples to what you may be feeling. It is your unique journey that is your real teacher. You have taught yourself how to heal. You have taught yourself how to take the first step, and you have taught yourself how to recognize greatness within yourself.

Are there people in your life who would be proud of you for where you are now? If so, you should greet them and share your renewed sense of pride and clarity with them. It is reaffirming of your own sense of accomplishments to have it validated by those you love, those you admire, and those you respect. Sometimes, it can give a new perspective to emphasize with someone else and share a joyful feeling with them. You are no longer in a cave of your own misjudgments, both internal and external. You have established yourself out in the light. You can walk among the world with your head high instead of living in the past and inside of your own head. You see the world for how it actually is and not through the lens of prior transgressions or feelings of worthlessness. It is even possible to look back at how you used to exist and treat yourself and separate yourself enough from it that you can even brush it off. That is not you anymore. You are the real you now. You are the you that you were meant to be, a much happier and more honest you who recognizes real emotions instead of perceived injustices to yourself.

Chapter 7: Living in the Positive!

Now that you have created a positive atmosphere for your mind to exist in, you are probably feeling a new motivation and longing to explore the world in your new self. What do you do with all of this motivation? It is important to put this good energy to use as to not fall back into negative habits that your old self has come to reinforce. You are at a crucial step where you should give great importance to channeling this positive energy into positive habits.

Something that you can do for yourself is to continue to practice meditation and exercise. Your new positive life starts at your core. Your core being yourself. You have learned a renewed sense of self-respect and discovered some deep insight into yourself. Now, it is time to maintain it. You can continue to live positive as long as you take care of yourself. Imagine yourself in a fancy car. It can look nice on the outside, but if the engine is not kept in good condition, it will not function as intended. Every new positive action starts with a sense of wellbeing.

Other ways to maintain your emotional stability through practice is to find a creative outlet for your feelings. If you feel that you are the creative type of person, then you may already have some of these hobbies. You may even have hobbies that you have not visited in a long time. Picking up an old hobby can help you connect with who you were before you found yourself down a darker path. It can give you a sense that you are picking up where you left off and reassure you that this you is the real you. If you are not a creative person or have not found an interest in a hobby, then do not worry! Another way that you can strengthen your mental focus and reinforce this new positive you are to learn. Reading is a proven method to increase cognitive faculties and helps you to directly discover interesting perspectives that you may not have come to on your own independently. Maybe, you will even discover ways to learn about aspects of your life that you have put on hold. Projects and promises made to others and you can now be fulfilled because you are now breathing easy and have a new motivation for life.

Great! Now that you have a healthy and positive sense of wellbeing, you can further reinforce your new positive life by engaging in productive social activities. Before I get into examples of this, I want to further explore the benefits.

Giving back to your community outwardly shows that you want to be engaged with society. You recognize yourself as a part of a whole and you are devoid of an ego that alienates you from your peers. It is not a struggle for your individuality though; you have already explored and defined yourself to yourself. Now, it is time to show who you are to the world! A person who lives inside of their own negative thought patterns does not want to be a part of society. They will build their own mental walls to keep themselves from embarrassment, anger, shame, or any other negative thought patterns associated with social interaction. Maybe they feel that society owes them something. An overinflated ego is another trepidation to avoid. Now that you are free of all of these negative thought patterns, you can enjoy social interaction with a head held high and nothing to apologize for. Another key benefit that you may not have seen or realized before, is that doing something nice for others simply feels good. You are able to emphasize the happiness of others. Seeing a smile on another person's face that you have caused can feel so rewarding in ways that you have never felt before! Even for more selfish reasons, it feels good, as in the sense of being the hero of someone's day. It is a wholesome feeling. It is a feeling that is entirely guilt-free. Some examples of positive social outings would be simple activities like volunteer work or attending or even participating in sports events. Maybe your place of employment has a softball league, or your colleagues enjoy disc golf. These are activities that directly give back to your community or peer group. These are higher levels of commitment, so if you are not ready for that quite yet, maybe you could try something a little less structured. Meeting trusted friends in a relaxed social environment could be a little bit more comfortable for you. Invite a friend, or a few friends, out for lunch or to a store of your common interests. This kind of setting makes for a good conversation that is not so personal if you are not ready for that. It is perfectly acceptable to take your time developing your social identity, as this step is very important. Meeting friends in this kind of setting can also help you learn more about your friends and even yourself! Maybe they have an interest that you did not even know that you had! Maybe you have a friend who is very interested in tabletop gaming, which might be an area of interest that you have never explored! Your friends and new interests will most likely lead you to new friends and even more positive and interesting activities. It is easy to get sucked into the positive life; all you have to do is take the first step!

Working within your comfortable level of commitment is essential, but it is also important to actually engage in these or similar activities. The goal of this section is to establish new positive habits to replace self-destructive habits. Just like how picking up and reading this book was a crucial first step, this is another crucial step. Do not fret though! This step is easier than what you would think. Most of the time, the fear associated with the activity is much worse than the actual activity, and you should know how to properly process negative thought patterns. All you have to do is breathe and take that step. Your friends, family, and colleagues will be more than happy to have you included.

It is important to establish positive relationships that engage in positive activities. It is also important to allow yourself to learn what positive social activities are. A common misconception, reinforced by advertisements and common television shows, is that all social activity takes place with alcohol. That is simply not true. In fact, the most productive and happiest people may rarely step foot in one of these establishments. As a side note, you may also be surprised at the money you save when you do not frequently visit these establishments, which brings me back to advertisements. That is why those media outlets pursue that lifestyle; it is purely to promote a lifestyle that will earn their company more money. In that respect, establish your own idea of happiness! Find out what it is that truly makes you happy! You are most likely to find that engaging with friends develops real bonds and promotes honest happiness. You are most likely to find that volunteer work, or even saying yes when someone asks for a favor, is more fulfilling than anything that you have experienced in your previous life.

You should feel proud of yourself for taking this step! Now that you are taking steps to not only better yourself, but to solidify and reinforce it with positive social activities, there is nothing that can get in your way on your path to being happier, more wholesome you! Once again, congratulations!

Chapter 8: How DBT Has Enhanced Your Life

Although this book has seemed to have an almost conversational flow, it has actually followed very closely to the five functions of DBT. As this book has mentioned before, the goal of this is not to assume an authoritative role over you, the reader. This book was designed to reinforce your own choices and merely give examples of positive living for those who may be unaware or fearful of how to live as such. Having said that, it is now time to relate what we have learned to the five functions of Dialectical Behavior Therapy. Before we do that, let's define what those five functions are.

- Enhance client's capabilities
- Improve the client's motivation
- Assure generalization to the client's natural environment
- Structure the environment
- Enhance the therapist's capabilities and support their motivation

The clinical way to go about enhancing your capabilities is to reinforce the skills of DBT. We have used many skills directly from the actual standard of DBT, such as the acronyms DEAR MAN, FAST, and PLEASE MASTER. These are acronyms that you would become familiar with if you were to attend a regular DBT session. We have also discussed important skills like practicing mindfulness and emotional regulation. These are also skills that you are most likely to encounter in an actual DBT session. This book has taken those lessons and broken them down for you to study, practice, and make into your own at your own pace by your own choices. Using these skills in your own life will only work to enhance the quality of your life and introduce you to lifestyles that mirror your interests, even those that you may not be aware that you have. This is an exciting time to be alive, and an exciting time for you!

The next function of DBT is the enhancement of the client's motivation. This book was designed to keep you motivated throughout, but it is not what was written or the speed in which you read it. The real motivation comes from you. You have rewarded yourself for picking up this book and sticking to it all the way to the end. By now, you deserve to have developed a sense of pride in making these positive changes in your life! There is no outside force that can motivate you to the extent that you can motivate yourself.

This book was written to be a companion to your own life. You are free to read or not read, follow or not follow, at your own pace. The fact that you have made it this far is something to be celebrated. It shows that you are honest in your desire to rid yourself of negative thought processes and self-destructive habits. There is not a single person or entity that is able to instill that level of motivation inside of you. You have shown that you are committed; not to this book or these processes, but you are committed to yourself. You have already taken better care of yourself than previously you might have thought possible. It is not only acceptable but appropriate to celebrate yourself at this time. This is a real achievement that you have accomplished, and one that many people take multiple tries to achieve. Some may not ever get to the level of clarity and health that you have already achieved for yourself. Once again, Congratulations!

The third function of DBT may seem confusing at first. It is to assure generalization to the client's natural environment. What that means is that this treatment, and this book, is designed to be a companion piece to live alongside without overtaking your life. This is not a program designed to put your life on hold. The effectiveness of this is that it promotes ease of transition into your new lifestyle while giving examples that are digestible by you because they relate to you, just as you are. It is easy to take this book with you and read it at your own pace or use the skills you have learned through a DBT session or in this book while you go about living your day-to-day life. There is no commitment besides the commitment that you have made to yourself and are comfortable with.

In an actual DBT session, they would address this function within the moment coaching. You would have access to a 24/7 phone number that you would be encouraged to call if you are having a hard time with applying the lessons to your life you would have learned during a session. This is an excellent tool, and if you were to attend a DBT session, I would strongly encourage you to feel free to use it. These coaches are not there to judge your choices. They understand the material and are also encouraged to process emotions without judgment. This is purely for the benefit of you! It is also encouraging to have outside motivation when your motivation might be hitting a low point. There is nothing to worry about though, just like the inevitability of sickness or negative thoughts, you cannot fault yourself for when your motivation is feeling weaker at the moment. Just relax, call that number, and celebrate yourself for making the positive choice at that moment when you may not have previously.

We are almost through the list here, I hope that you feel encouraged to continue. The fourth function of DBT is to structure the client's environment. This one can seem almost scary because you have gone this far along your own choices. There is nothing to fear though because this step is not designed to take away your choices, merely to help you and provide tools for you to make positive choices when you may not have previously. How a DBT session would go about doing that would be to assign you a case manager. This is someone who is dedicated to your case and is working with you to ensure your success.

An important aspect of this function is the thought process when accepting it. It is not there to control your lifestyle. When a client has made poor life choices and made a habit out of them, then they might not be aware of or be comfortable with lifestyle choices that are more positive and sustainable. You have already decided to live a positive life, now it is time to learn how. That is the purpose of this function. In DBT, there is a strong focus on replacing negative habits with more positive habits. This is because pure motivation has to be outwardly expressed and used for it to continue. Imagine your positive motivation as a match. You can light the match, and it will burn for a while. It is hot, it is bright. It has the potential to continue on, but it can only continue on if fuel is introduced to the match. Imagine this function of DBT as a pile of wood arranged for you in a fire pit, ready to be lit by your motivational match. Once you apply the match to the wood in the fire pit, then the fire burns much longer in a safe environment. Your motivation must be applied to a positive atmosphere to continue on. Your case manager or other individuals in your DBT session use this function to safely provide you with those structured, positive environments. Go forth and do well for yourself and others!

Have you made it this far? I hope that you have because this is now the final function of Dialectical Behavior Therapy. That function is to enhance the therapist's capabilities and support their motivation. DBT therapists work in a team to more effectively enhance the lives and understanding of their clients. This is important for the team as well as the client. A typical DBT team meeting may start with a mindfulness exercise, reading of the previous minutes, and then discuss strategies to further their treatment. It is important for you to be engaging and helpful along with your therapist as this whole treatment only works with your commitment. An example of this would be to imagine you and your therapist on a rowboat. Your therapist will not be able to motivate you to continue to row if they are not participating in the work. Your therapist can also not row by themselves if you are not helping. This whole style of treatment is designed to be a cooperative endeavor. You should feel excited and encouraged to participate. The end result will be a happier, more positive you!

This chapter is here to serve the purpose of relating what you have learned to the structured skills that are discussed in an actual Dialectical Behavior Therapy session. It is strongly encouraged that you attend these sessions and take what you have learned in this book with you to those sessions. There is nothing that you should not be able to achieve in this aspect of your life between this book, those sessions, and your own motivation! You have a threefold angle of attack on your negative habits that you wish to eradicate from your life. Finding a DBT session is easy, as it is a growing style of treatment. Everyone involved wishes only the best of success for you! Continue on with your own choices and feel proud of how far you have come!

PART IV

Chapter 1: Energy Healing- The Key to Holistic Health

Understanding the impacts of energy imbalances and corresponding physical, mental, spiritual health

How many times have you, or another adult in your life, said the words "I just don't have the energy I used to have."? Most adults know the feeling of looking at the energy children have as they run about, enjoying life, exploring their surroundings, and never seeming to grow tired. Many of us are left reflecting back on the distance past when we, too, had such energy, and wondering where it went.

From the time children enter school, they begin to be presented with expectations. Stand in a straight line, raise your hand, don't talk while the teacher is talking. Each year, the level of responsibility and expectation seems to increase. While rules, regulations, and individual responsibility are important for a functioning society, there are numerous expectations and social pressures put on people as they grow which can be incredibly harmful.

It is generally around middle school when children become more acutely aware of their bodies and societal beauty standards which tell them what they "should" look like. Children are likely to become aware of the trends, such as which clothes the "cool kids" are wearing. The endless battle to feel like enough begins, and can lead to a plethora of issues with self-esteem, eating disorders, and mental illness. In addition to the basic societal pressures to be accepted and considered attractive, many children are also faced with difficult situations at home where their own needs are not being met, they are having to provide for and protect themselves in the only ways they know how, avoid abusive parents, care for younger siblings, or worry about if they'll have anything to eat that day. Even if children have a relatively healthy home life, this is the age when they will begin to become aware of the issues that plague their family (every family has issues) whether this is divorce, an alcoholic parent, the death of a pet or loved one, etc.

We live in a society which thrives off of consumerism. We are flooded with images of how the next vacation, new pair of shoes, nicer car, nicer house, or perfect partner will make us happy, and all of the things we need to change about ourselves in order to fulfill those things. Eventually, all the energy we had as a child starts going towards maintaining our image in society, trying to have all the "best" life has to offer (which always happens to be everything we do not have), and attempting to be as "successful" as possible in the eyes of society and other people. With no time to rest in the present moment, recharge, and appreciate what we already have, it is no wonder so many of us are completely drained of energy. In such a fast-paced society that discourages breaks, our energy will become depleted and we will find ourselves thrown out of balance and unable to obtain true happiness and well-being. Overtime, this depletion and imbalance can lead to a sense of spiritual disconnection, extreme mental health issues, and an increased risk of physical pain, illness, and even earlier death.

Chapter 2: Energy Healing and Overcoming Suffering

Energy and Grief/Trauma

Every human being knows that loss is a natural part of life. The one certain thing in life is that we, and everyone we know, is going to die. However, in such a fast-paced society, we are often given a very short grace period before being expected to swallow our grief and "move on" when we lose those closest to us. It is not abnormal for people to receive a bereavement period of only a few days before being expected to be back in the classroom or office and be fully functional. There is very little space for the grief journey, and most people are expected to harbor their feelings and keep their grief to themselves.

The grief process is expansive and incredibly energy draining. When we don't receive the adequate support from those around us, or adequate space to heal, our body begins to break down piece by piece. The empty spaces within us will swallow us up into states of depression, numbness, isolation, and pure exhaustion. Just like a wound being denied the correct treatment and care, the wounds of unresolved grief will fester and leave us feeling completely drained of energy and vitality for life.

Unresolved trauma also has an incredibly destructive impact on the body. Trauma can occur as a result of grief itself, as well as emotional or domestic abuse, accident or illness, war, sexual assault, childhood maltreatment, etc. The body holds trauma in various places, and the brain switches over from the logical ability to discern safety and danger into an easily triggered emotional state. An overactive emotional brain loses the ability to think clearly, make decisions, and recognize threats. People who have unresolved trauma are likely to be easily triggered and deal with unexplained outbursts of anger, fear, relationship issues, reckless behavior, and health problems. When trauma sits in the body unresolved, the brain is unable to understand that the traumatic event has ended. Therefore, it will stay in a consistent fight-or-flight state, which is incredibly draining and will leave the body with no energy. Not only will trauma victims experience low energy levels, they will also experience severe issues maintaining positive relationships and overall well-being.

Energy and Mental Health

There are numerous factors which can contribute to mental health issues.

As previously discussed, societal issues and unresolved grief and trauma can yield higher levels of anxiety, depression, and PTSD. It is also very common for people to suffer from mood disorders, personality disorders, disordered eating, substance abuse, etc. The list is long for psychological ailments and how they happen, and it has been proven that 1 in 3 people will be diagnosed with a mental illness in their lifetime. Even without a specific disorder, most people will have periods of life where their mental health suffers greatly.

No matter what a person's struggle with mental health looks like, or what they are doing (or not doing) in terms of treatment, the body expends a lot of energy when a part of it is unwell.

Daily Energy Regulation

No matter what it is in your life that is causing you to feel depleted, it is vital to pay attention to the energy fields within the body and identify the areas of greatest pain and imbalance. In the spectrum of health, people often take measures such as going to see the doctor, therapist, or grief counselor, taking medication, and making lifestyle changes such as finding a hobby or increasing exercise. However, a piece that is commonly overlooked in the healing journey is healing energetically. No matter how much you invest in your mental, physical, emotional, and spiritual health, if your energies remain imbalanced, it is impossible to reach a state of full wellness. That being said, energy healing is the missing piece in most people's quests for holistic health.

In many cases, it can be beneficial to seek the help of energy healers, massage therapists, and reiki, craniosacral therapy, or bodywork practitioners. These practitioners are trained in getting in touch with your energy centers and helping bring them back into balance through healing touch, body movements, and visualization techniques. If you are dealing with energy imbalance, seeing a practitioner can be an excellent investment in unlocking your highest levels of health and joy in life.

It is also possible to use a variation of the body scan mediation from chapter 3 to check in with your energy levels on your own. By taking notice of the sensations in each area of your body, you can come closer in touch with any area of your body where you experience regular pain, tension, or other unpleasant feelings. This is often a sign of imbalance or trapped energy. Additionally, the tense and release technique in each area of the body can yield healing and balance by releasing negative energy and tension. It is important to check in with yourself daily, asking your body where energy may be trapped or depleted and what you can do to replenish yourself.

Chapter 3: The Daily Energy Healing Journey

Understanding Your Energy Field: Daily Energy Healing Meditation with Journaling (Week 5)

There is great variety when it comes to human energy fields. People experience varying levels of sensitivity to the energy of other people and the environment. Some people are incredibly in tune with "vibes", others are empaths who feel the emotional experiences of others on a deep level, while still others experience very little of either. There is also a lot of variation in the way people recharge energetically, as well as what depletes them. In the common case of introverts and extroverts, for example, introverts need time alone to replenish their energy and feel balanced, while extroverts recharge in stimulating environments with other people around. One of the first steps to protecting your personal energetic field is to understand how it works.

Understanding Your Energy Field Journal Prompt (Week 5):

When you feel exhausted and not like yourself, which activities are most likely to replenish your energy? Do you enjoy a night out with friends? Yoga? A walk in the park? Leisure reading? Finding a new adventure? Taking a bubble bath? Listening to your favorite music on blast? List 5-10 activities which help you gain balance and feel energized.

Now, make a list of the things that make you feel most drained. These can be large things, like a specific task at your job, or small things like doing the dishes. You may find that you feel drained if you spend too much time alone or, consequently, when you spend too much time around other people.

When it comes to activities that make you feel drained, ask yourself to what extent that specific thing is necessary in your life. If you find yourself feeling drained from spending too much time around other people, for example, you can easily make a change by scheduling more "nothing time" or "alone time" into your days and taking the time you need to replenish. Household tasks and daily responsibilities are necessary, but by being aware of the ones that drain you the most, you can bring more attention into the process and doing what you need to replenish energy before or after.

Protecting Your Energy Field: Daily Energy Healing Meditation with Journaling (Week 6)

Close your eyes and ask yourself "what does my energy field look like?" Write down any specific colors, textures, shapes, or patterns of movement.

Once you have an image in your mind of your energy field, ask yourself "What does it look like for outside energies to enter my field?" Write down what healthy and unhealthy outside energies look like.

Then ask yourself "How can I regulate the energies entering my field? What does it look like when I decide what I will let in?" Describe this process.

Finally, ask yourself "How does my body feel when I regulate what I allow to enter my energy field?" Write down everything that comes to mind.

Healing Through Trapped Emotion Release: Daily Energy Healing Meditation with Journaling (Week 7)

In our society, we are often faced with life circumstances that force us to repress our basic human emotions. It is very possible for anger, rage, or grief to become stuck in the body because it is considered "impractical" to have those reactions in public. Similarly, we often hear about people being described as "annoyingly happy" or "overly emotional." Most of us are taught not only to manage our emotions, but to distance ourselves from them and react emotionally only in certain contexts. Additionally, we tend to suppress negative emotions such as fear, shame, inadequacy, and insecurity, for the purpose of appearing like we have everything together. Between life events and societal expectations, it is very easy for the emotions we suppress to become trapped in our bodies, which can create adverse health effects, negatively impact our relationships, and keep us from living our best lives.

Begin by making a list of as many emotions as you can think of

Run down the list of emotions one by one, asking yourself "Is there anywhere in my body I am holding *particular emotion*?"

Write down the emotions you feel are trapped. Take some time to journal about how certain emotions arose, or times when you felt you had to suppress your emotions.

With each emotion you have labeled as being trapped, write: "I give myself permission to release this *particular emotion*

Cultivating Self-Trust in your Healing Journey: Daily Energy Healing Meditation with Journaling (Week 8)

No matter what you do in your life, there will always be people who don't understand the choices you make, or who judge the path you are on. When it comes to renewing and protecting your energy, there is no room for anyone else's opinions or emotions in regards to your journey. It requires a great deal of self-trust to go your own way and let what other people think about it roll off your back. For this reason, it is vital to begin everyday establishing a sense of self-trust with your own journey and energy management skills. The following four journal questions will help you direct your energy before going about your day.

What are you most grateful for today?

What are your intentions for how you will direct your energy today?

What are your fears/things you perceive as a potential threat?

What are your commitments to yourself and the world?

Mini Meditation Toolbox: 25 Quick and Easy Energy Restoration and Protection Meditations

One-Minute Energy Cleanse

- This meditation is useful if you find yourself with a person or in a specific situation that feels negative or energetically draining. You do not need to be alone to complete this meditation

- Pause where you are and allow yourself to take a few deep, cleansing breaths

- Focus exclusively on your breathing; you may close your eyes or leave them open

- Feel the inner power within the core of your body, around your abdomen. Remind yourself that you are in control and have the power to maintain balance.

- As you inhale, pull love, light, and peace into your body

- As you exhale, breathe out pain, annoyance, and toxicity

Energy from the Earth

- Begin by entering a space in nature. This can be on the beach, in the mountains, near a river, in a garden, by the lake, or in your own yard

- If possible, slip your shoes off so your bare feet are in contact with the earth

- Start with a few cleansing breaths, taking note of everything you see, hear, smell, and feel in your environment

- Placing the soles of your feet on the ground, begin to breathe, pulling the energy from the earth up through your body

- Remember that you are One with the nature that courses around you. Allow it to heal what is broken within you and leave you feeling rejuvenated

Re-Centering Head Hold (3-5 minute meditation)

- Close your eyes and place the palm of one hand horizontally across the crown of your head, and the other palm across your forehead (over the energetic points of the Crown and Third Eye chakras). This position can be done while standing, sitting, or lying down.

- While clutching your head in this position, bring attention to any sensations in your body. What needs your attention most right now?

- Allow yourself to come back to the present moment, feeling grounded in your body and in your experience

- Breathe in awareness, focus, and comfort, exhaling anxiety and distraction

- When you open your eyes, notice how you feel grounded in your space

The Cloak of Protection

- This meditation is useful for energy protection before going out in to the world, whether that is to work, the supermarket, an appointment, etc.

- Although you do not know what kinds of energies you may encounter, or which people may try to take your energy from you, remind yourself that you are in control of your own energy and that you have the capacity to protect yourself

- Close your eyes and imagine a dark-blue, almost black cloak made of soft, thick material like a velvet night sky. The cloak is full-length with a hood to protect all of your chakras.

- Imagine a ray of light outlining the cloak in whatever color(s) feel most magical, protective, and authentic to who you are

- Set off into the world knowing that you are safe within yourself and your energy cloak, and that you do not need to be afraid

De-Cluttering your Space

- When energy is lacking or out of balance, the spaces we live in are likely to reflect that imbalance with clutter and messiness. The more we feel like we "don't have our lives together", the more likely we are to have a messy desk, dishes piling up in the sink, laundry that still needs to be folded, or a car that has not been cleared of trash

- Such spaces do not allow for peace and mental clarity, and can be even more draining to come back to after a long day

- Dedicate yourself to one area of your life to de-clutter. This can be your kitchen, your car, your bedroom, etc. Close your eyes before beginning and take a few deep, cleansing breaths to approach the task calmly

- Begin to address all of the clutter in the space, not only picking it up, but putting it into a designated area where it can be organized and easy to find

- You may find that you want to create a special shelf or move some furniture around to make the space less cluttered. As you go, notice the energy that continues to unfold in your body

- When you finish, place a "clutter basket" in your room, the car, the living room, etc. where you can compile all the clutter throughout the day and put it away before bed

De-Cluttering your Mind (5-minute meditation)

- Close your eyes and begin to breathe deeply

- Ask yourself "What is taking up the most space in my mind right now?"

- Bring your attention to whatever it is that is distracting you, and why it makes you feel out of control

- Breathe into that situation, saying "I have control over this situation, and I am not going to let it spill out into the rest of my day. I am clearing this space."

The Energy-Ownership Mantra

- This meditation is ideal to perform in the morning, or before going out to interact with the world or other people

- Sit in a place where you feel energized (on the porch, in your meditation corner, etc.)

- Close your eyes and begin to breathe, checking in with any unresolved emotions or senses within the body

- Now begin to picture your energy field. Say to yourself: "My energy field is my sacred space, and other energies will only permeate it when I allow them to."

- Breathe into this thought for several moments

- Now, bring this thought into your mental space: "I have the wisdom to discern what belongs to me and what belongs to other people. I can be empathetic and attentive to other people's emotions, struggles, and opinions, without assuming responsibility for them."

Epsom Bath Energy Renewal

- Begin by selecting your favorite scented Epsom salts. You may also customize your bath with petals, oils, and candles as according to the healing plants, herbs, and oils listed in Chapter 4

- Run a hot bath, letting your Epsom salts and other elements saturate the water

- Customize your space with the light of candles, meditative music, and anything else that makes you feel at peace

- Find a comfortable position inside the tub. Close your eyes, and feel your entire body relax into the heat and gentle movement of the water.

- Begin to conduct a body scan, feeling entirely vulnerable to this moment at peace with only yourself

- Ask your body "What do I need right now?"

- The water should be hot enough that you begin to sweat (be sure to have a glass of water nearby). As you sweat, imagine your body purging itself of every blockage, every impurity, and every negativity

Sealing your Energy Field

- Close your eyes and begin to breathe

- Bring the image of your energy field to your mind. You may picture a wall, a bubble, or a glowing ring of light (this image may also differ depending on the day)

- Picture what other energies look like, floating around your field like particles in an atom. Say to yourself "I am in control of what comes in."

- Imagine yourself recognizing people who are trying to take your energy or bear their burdens. Imagine any fear, anger, or resentment you may feel.

- Say to yourself "No, not today." Imagine your bubble becoming impermeable, your wall being sealed, your glowing ring of light rejecting anything that does not belong inside

- Allow yourself to feel empowered over your energy, without feeling any resentment or judgment towards those who once posed a threat

Building your Sanctuary

- Sit down and close your eyes, beginning to breathe into yourself

- With each breath, ask yourself "What makes me feel safe?" Repeat three times.

- Switch the phrase to "What makes me feel at peace?" Repeat three times.

- Switch the phrase to "What makes me feel loving?" Repeat three times

- Switch to "What makes me feel joy?"

- Lastly, ask yourself "What makes me feel renewed?"

- When you ask yourself these questions, you may see certain crystals, scenes in nature, types of music, plants, aromas, decorations, activities, or color schemes. Take note of whatever comes to mind.

- Use these things that come to you in meditation to mindfully cultivate a space for yourself to come into every day when you need time to recharge. This can be a meditation corner, a spot in the backyard, or any other space that is sacred to you and provides feelings of security and rest.

Cultivating Non-Reaction

- This meditation can be used when encountering a stressful situation, having a difficult conversation, or otherwise entering a state of nervous or angry energy

- Before responding to whatever the negative stimulant is, breathe into the moment. Close your eyes if needed.

- Tell yourself "I can choose not to expend energy on this interaction. I can choose to move peacefully into the next moment."

- Feel the tension within you melt away as you make the choice not to internalize the stress of the situation or the negative energy coming at you

Boundary Setting

- Find a quiet place to sit and self-reflect. Breathe into the moment

- After you have settled into your breath, ask yourself "What people, circumstances, or tasks drain my energy and leave me feeling agitated or exhausted?"

- Allow the answers to rise into your consciousness at will. Meditate on every name, every task, every circumstance which makes you feel tense and throws your energy out of balance.

- With each name, circumstance, and task, say to yourself "This *person, place, thing* has no power over me. I can maintain my energy in spite of it."

- Next, ask yourself "Where do I need to draw the line with this *person, place, thing*?"

- Listen to your intuition tell you what your boundaries should be. Perhaps, this looks like gently cutting off a toxic person, or limiting your interaction time with them. It could be quitting a job that is no longer good for you, or asking for accommodations to make your environment more positive. It could be telling someone who expects you to bear their burdens that their energies are no longer your responsibility. Or, perhaps it is to establish a self-care activity to do directly after a draining task.

Trigger Awareness

- If your energy has ever been thrown out of balance by trauma, there are likely still factors of your environment which can strike at any time, causing your body to react in the same way it did at the time of the trauma.

- Breathe into the moment, asking yourself "what elements of my environment cause me to lose control of my logic and feel afraid, helpless, irrational, in pain, or otherwise unbalanced or unhealthy energetically"

- These elements are called "triggers." Bring your awareness to these triggers, simply allowing them to be there without judgment.

- Say to yourself "that moment in time is over. I can now release myself."

Energetic Tapping

- Begin by determining 3-5 affirmations or manifestations for the day ahead ("I manifest peace," "I am content," "I am present," "I manifest energy," "I am growing," "I manifest healing," "I manifest loving-kindness", etc.)

- Breathe deeply, pondering the affirmations/manifestations

- Choose your first manifestation/affirmation. With your index and middle fingers on both hands, begin tapping lightly on the crown of your head, repeating the manifestation or affirmation three times

- Move to the temples, tapping and saying the manifestation/affirmation three times

- Repeat at the inner corners of the brow bone

- Repeat just above the brow line

- Repeat at the top of the cheek bones

- Repeat below the ear lobes at the crest of the jawbone

- Repeat at the top of the chest

- Repeat on the left wrist, then switch to right wrist

- Switch to the next affirmation/manifestation and go through the process again, staying in touch with your breath throughout

Listening to your Intuition

- Find a space where you feel completely comfortable and relaxed

- Begin to breathe deeply, coming into the present moment

- Ask yourself "What does my inner self need me to know right now?"

- Keep breathing, holding space for whatever answer arises

- If necessary, you can ask follow-up questions to yourself like "Is there any threat I need to be prepared to protect myself from?" or "How can I best love the world today?" Or "What do I need to do to take care of myself today?"

- Continue to breathe and hold space, trusting that your heart will guide you to make the correct decisions for yourself

Memory Reclamation (specifically for healing of trauma victims)

- Find a space where you feel totally safe and undisturbed. It is best to do this meditation on a day where you can invest in self-care and rest.

- Begin to breathe, telling yourself "I am safe. I am safe. I am safe."

- Allow the memory of a particularly traumatic event to come to your mind. Continue to breathe, telling yourself "I am safe."

- Pay attention to the details of that memory. What do you see? What do you hear? What do you feel?

- As the memory progresses, allow it to release its energetic hold on your body. Tell yourself "That was then. This is now. I am safe."

- Feel the trauma release its hold on you, restoring itself to a basic memory of the past

Defining your Needs

- Sit in a peaceful place, breathing into the moment

- Bring attention to any pain or unrest within your body. Without judgment, allow it to be there, asking if there is anything you should learn from it.

- Generally, where there is pain or unrest, there is a need being left unmet. Ask yourself "What is it that I need?"

- Allow your needs to arise into your consciousness ("I need a day off for my mental health," "I need a trip into nature," "I need a bath," "I need a warm, nourishing meal," "I need to go to sleep early," etc.)

- Breathe into each need, envisioning yourself meeting that particular need

- Ask yourself "Is there anyone else I need to make aware of these needs?"

- Envision yourself having a calm conversation about your needs with your boss, your partner, your family, or a friend. Envision them reacting gently and yourself feeling better understood and supported.

- Continue to breathe into your capacity to meet your energetic needs and make those needs known to others.

"Nothing Time"

- Set aside a minimum of one hour of time with absolutely nothing scheduled

- Sit down, breathing into the moment. Tell yourself "this is my time. I have nowhere to be, nothing to do, I do not need to feel rushed."

- Allow your deepest intuition to guide your next step. Do whatever comes to mind first

- While you proceed with your "nothing time", allow your breath to guide every move

Discovering your Support System

- Bring your attention to the present moment, focusing on your breath

- Ask yourself "Who of the people I know understands and embraces me for who I truly am?"

- Breathe with each name that comes up, allowing loving-kindness and appreciation for that person to flow through your body

- Ask yourself "Who in my life encourages me to reach my full potential?

- Repeat the action of breathing with each name that arises

- Ask yourself "Who in my life do I feel most at rest with?"

- Repeat the action of breathing with each name that arises

- Continue to breathe, saying to yourself "These are my people. This is my support system. I will allow myself to lean on them when I need to."

Glowing Love-Energy

- Find a restful position and begin to breathe

- Imagine the aura of your energy field. How big is it? What color is it?

- Say to yourself "I am pure love. I have room to love the entire universe and everything in it."

- Continue to repeat this phrase with every breath. Picture the aura expanding and glowing brighter

Jaguar Spirit Animal Protection

- Bring yourself into the present moment with deep breathing

- From the depth of your being, say "I call on the spirit of the jaguar to protect me."

- Feel the reverberations of the jaguar's protection through your body, aiding you in repelling negative energy and toxicity

- Imagine a fierce, beautiful guard of your energy field, encircling you with fierce love and security

Energetic Breathing (1-3-minute meditation)

- Take some space away from your everyday life (in the bathroom, in the car, etc.) to just breathe

- Implement the 5-5-7 breathing technique

- With every breath in, say to yourself, "I breathe in pure energy."

- With every breathe out, say to yourself, "I breathe out *exhaustion, *toxicity, *negativity, etc."

- Continue until you feel the tingle of pure energy coursing through your veins

Energetic Dancing/Movement

- Find a space where you can be alone and feel completely secure

- Play a song that stirs your soul and emotions, causing you to have a visceral reaction in the body each time you hear it

- As the song begins, close your eyes and deep breathe, maybe swaying back and forth slightly

- When you feel ready, release your body to move as it feels led. No choreography, no expectations, simply letting the movement of the moment lead your body into a state of pure surrender and release

- Surrender entirely to the moment, trusting your body to release any tension or trauma

- Give your body the space and freedom to heal, coming into energetic harmony

The Art of Saying "No"

- Close your eyes and begin to breathe deeply

- Begin to consider the things that drain your energy. Perhaps you have a tendency to overcommit, or find yourself stuck in a relationship or circumstance that no longer serves you. Breathe with each of these places where you feel stuck

- Say to yourself "I have the power to say 'no.'"

- Imagine yourself having the necessary conversation, turning down the opportunity, or simply choosing to remove yourself from the situation

- Feel the power of saying no and being in full control of where you place your energy

The Restorative Power of Letting Go

- Breathe deeply, cultivating a sense of full peace and security

- Ask yourself "Where are the parts of me that I need to get back?"

- Take notice of every person or place that comes to mind as still having a part of your energy and your essence

- If there are any feelings of melancholy, nostalgia, resentment, shame, or anger, allow them to be there, breathing as they flow through you

- Say to yourself "I release this *person or place*. I reclaim what they have that is rightfully mine."

- Continue to breathe into this empowerment

PART V

Chapter 1: Self-Care Is the Best Care

"It is so important to take time for yourself and find clarity. The most important relationship is the one you have with yourself."

-Diane Von Furstenberg

Self-care is any activity that we deliberately do to improve our own well-being, whether it is physical, emotional, mental, or spiritual. The importance of taking care of one's self cannot be denied, as even health care training focuses on making sure healthcare workers are caring for themselves. If you do not take care of yourself, eventually, every other aspect o your life will fall apart, including your ability to help others.

This is a very simple concept, yet it is highly overlooked in the grand scheme of things. People lack the tendency to look after themselves and put their needs before anyone else. Good self-care is essential to improving our mood and reducing our anxiety levels. It will do wonders for reducing exhaustion and burnout, which is very common in our fast-paced world. It will also lead to positive improvements in our relationships.

One thing to note is that self-care does not mean forcing ourselves to do something we don't like, no matter how enjoyable it is to other people. For example, if your friends are forcing you to go to a party you rather not attend, then giving in is not taking care of yourself. If you would rather stay in and watch a movie, then that's what you should do, and it will be better for your well-being.

How Does Self-Care Work

It is difficult to pinpoint exactly what self-care is, as it is personal for everybody. Some people love to pamper themselves by going to the spa, while others enjoy physical activities like hiking, biking, or swimming. Some individuals take up art or other hobbies, like writing or playing a musical instrument. These activities are all different but will have the same type of benefits for the individuals engaging in them.

The main factor to consider when engaging in self-care is to determine if you enjoy the activity in question. If not, then it's time to move on. Self-care is an active choice that you actually have to plan out. It is time you set aside for yourself to make sure all of your needs are met. If you use a planner of any sort, make sure to dedicate some space for your particular self-care activities. Also, let people who need to know about your plans so you can become more committed. Pay special attention to how you feel afterward. The objective of any self-care activity is to make yourself feel better. If this is not happening, then it's time to change the activity.

While self-care, as a whole, is individualized, there is a basic checklist to consider.

- Create a list of things you absolutely don't want to do during the self-care process. For instance, not checking emails, not answering the phone,

avoiding activities you don't enjoy, or not going to specific gatherings, like a house party.
- Eat nutritious and healthy meals most of the time, while indulging once in a while.
- Get the proper amount of sleep according to your needs.
- Avoid too many negative things, like news or social media.
- Exercise regularly.
- Spend appropriate time with your loved ones. These are the people you genuinely enjoy and not forced relationships.
- Look for opportunities to enjoy yourself and laugh.
- Do at least one relaxing activity a day, like taking a bath, going for a walk, or cooking a meal.

Self-care is extremely important and should not be an anomaly in your life.

How Does Self-Care Improve Self-Esteem and Self-Confidence?

To bring everything full circle, self-care plays a major role in improving self-esteem and self-confidence. It is easy to see how taking care of yourself will also make you feel better about yourself overall. All of these are actually inter-related, and a lack of one showcases a lack of the other. While caring for yourself also improves your self-esteem and self-confidence, not having self-esteem or self-confidence also leads to a lack of self-care. Basically, you believe that you are not good enough to be taken care of.

People with high self-esteem and self-confidence value themselves as much as they value others, and have no issues with making sure they're taken care of. They realize that it does not make them selfish or inconsiderate to think in this manner. Even if other people try to make them feel that way, a self-confident person will just brush off the criticism. An important thing to note is that when you take care of yourself, it does not mean you don't care about other people. It simply means you have enough self-love to not place yourself on the backburner.

Many people work so hard to try and please everyone else. This is one of the telltale signs of low self-esteem. While they're busy worried about other peoples' needs, their own get neglected, which will wear them down over time. The more they're unable to please someone, the harder they will try. What people in this situation don't realize is that some people are impossible to please, and it is not their responsibility to please them. That is up to the individual.

Poor self-care will eventually lead to poor self-image. It is possible that a person already has this initially. Self-care includes taking care of your hygienic and grooming needs. If you don't take the time to make yourself look good, this will significantly impact the value you place on yourself. When you are t work, among your friends, or just walking around town, not feeling like you look good will ultimately make you feel like you don't belong anywhere. Your confidence levels will plummet due to this.

Your health is another aspect to consider. Poor self-care means bad sleeping habits, unhealthy diets, lack of exercise, and more self-destructive behaviors. Your poor health practices can result in chronic illnesses down the line, like heart disease or diabetes. Once again, diminished health will lead to reduced self-confidence and self-esteem. Ask yourself now if putting other people ahead of you is worth it? I've got some news for you. The people who demand the most from you are probably looking out for themselves first.

The less a person takes care of themselves, the more their self-esteem and self-confidence will decline. It turns into a vicious downward cycle. This is why it is important to focus on all of these areas equally. When you find yourself neglecting your own self-care practices, it is time to shift your direction and bring your attention back to your needs. Ignoring your needs will ultimately lead to your fall. We will discuss specific practices and techniques for improving self-care in the next chapter.

Chapter 2:

What Does Good Self-Care Look Like?

Good Self-Care Practices

The following are some ways that good self-care will look like. If you find yourself having these qualities, then you are on the right path.

Taking Responsibility for Your Happiness
When you engage in self-care, it is truly self-care. This means you only rely on yourself, and nobody else, to make sure your needs are met. You realize that your happiness is no one else's responsibility but your own. You alone have the ability to control your outcomes. As a result of this independence, you will develop the skills and attitude you need to care for your own physical, mental, emotional, and spiritual well-being.

You Become Assertive With Others
People often take assertiveness for rudeness. This is not true, but if people believe that standing firm for what you want is rude, then that's their problem. Once you reach a certain mindset where self-care is important to you, then you will be unapologetically assertive. This means you have the ability to say "no" with confidence and stand by it. "No" is a complete sentence, and people will realize that quickly when they hear it from you.

You Treat Yourself As You Would a Close Friend
It's interesting how we believe that other people deserve better treatment from us than we do ourselves. We have a tendency to put our best friends in front of

us, no matter how detrimental it is to our lives. This behavior stops once we engage in proper self-care. At this point, you will treat yourself as good as, or even better, than you treat your most beloved friends.

You Are Not Afraid to Ask for What You Want

Once you learn to take care of yourself, you also see your value increase within your mind. This means having an understanding that your voice, opinion, and needs matter, just like anybody with high self-esteem and self-confidence, would. As a result, you will not be afraid to ask for what you want, even if you might not get it.

Your Life Is Set Around Your Own Values

Once you practice self-care, you learn to check in with yourself before making important decisions. You always make sure the choices you are about to make line up with your purpose and values. If they go against them, then it's not a path you choose. This goes for the career you choose, where you decide to live, and the relationships you maintain in your life.

While all of the traits are focused on self, but it will lead to better relationships with other people too. When you practice self-care, you are in a better state in every aspect of your being. This gives you the ability to take care of and help those you need you, as well. Self-care is not an option, but a necessity, and it must never be ignored. Taking care of yourself is not selfish, no matter what anybody tells you. If someone tries to make you feel guilty over this matter, then consider distancing or removing them from your life. You are not obligated to maintain relationships with people.

Chapter 3: Demanding Your Own Self-Care

We went over the importance of self-care, and now we will focus on making it a reality in your life. If you want self-care to occur, you must be willing to demand it. The world is full of people who expect you to be at there beck-and-call every moment of the day. Some of these individuals are those who are closest to us, like friends or family members. This can make it harder to make our demands heard, but there is no way around it. Taking care of yourself is not an idea you can budge on. It is extremely important. We will go over several ways to maintain your ability for self-care in your life and provide detailed action steps to help you progress in this area.

Setting Healthy Boundaries

One of the biggest obstacles to self-care is other people who surround you. These are the true selfish individuals, whether they realize it or not, who believe they can barge in on your life and deserve all of your attention. They will take advantage of you, and if you are not careful, they will completely gain control of your emotions, and even your life. For proper self-care to occur, you must set firm and healthy boundaries with people. The following are steps that need to become mainstays in your life.

Identify and Name Your Limits
You must understand what your emotional, physical, mental, and spiritual limits are. If you do not know, then you will never be able to set real boundaries with people. Determine what behaviors you can tolerate and accept, and then consider what makes you feel uncomfortable. Identifying and separating these traits will

help us determine our lines.

Stay Tuned Into Your Feelings

Two major emotions that are red flags that indicate a person is crossing a barrier are resentment or discomfort. Whenever you are having these feelings, it is important to determine why. Resentment generally comes from people taking advantage of us or feelings of being unappreciated. In this instance, we are likely pushing ourselves beyond our limits because we feel guilty. Guilt-trips is a weapon that many people use to get their way. It is important to recognize when someone is trying to make you feel guilty because they are way overstepping their boundaries. Resentment could also be due to someone imposing their own views or values onto us. When someone makes you feel uncomfortable, that is another indication of a boundary crossed. Stay in tune with both of these emotions.

Don't Be Afraid of Being Direct

With some people, setting boundaries is easy because they have a similar communication style. They can simply read your cues and back off when needed. For other individuals, a more direct approach is needed. Some people just don't get the hint that they've crossed a line. You must communicate to them in a firm way that they have crossed your limits, and you need some space. A respectful person will honor your wishes without hesitation. If they don't, then that's on them. Your personal space is more important than their feelings.

Give Yourself Permission to Set Boundaries

The potential downfalls to personal limits are fear, self-doubt, and guilt. We may fear the other person's response when we set strong boundaries. Also, we may feel guilty if they become emotional about it. We may even have self-doubt on whether we can maintain these limits in the long run. Many individuals have the mindset that in order to be a good daughter, son, parent, or friend, etc., we have to say "yes" all the time. They often wonder if they deserve to have boundaries and limits with those closest to them. The answer is, yes, you do. You need to give yourself permission to set limits with people because they are essential to maintaining healthy relationships too. Boundaries are also a sign of self-respect. Never feel bad for respecting yourself.

Consider Your Past and Present

Determine what roles you have played throughout your life in the various relationships you have had. Were you the one who was always the caretaker? If so, then your natural tendency may be to put others before yourself. Also, think about your relationships now. Are you the one always taking care of things, or is it a reciprocal relationship? For example, are you always the one making plans, buying gifts, having dinner parties, and being responsible for all of the important aspects of the relationships? If this is the case, then tuning into your needs is especially important here. If you are okay with the dynamics of the relationship, then that's fine. I can't tell you how to feel. However, if you feel anger and resentment over this, then it's time to let your feeling be known, unapologetically.

Be Assertive

Once again, this does not mean being rude, even though some people will interpret it that way. Being assertive simply means being firm, which is important when reminding someone about your boundaries. Creating boundaries alone is not enough. You also have to stand by them and let people know immediately if they've crossed them. Let the person know in a respectful but strong tone that you are uncomfortable with where they're going, and they need to give you some space. Assertive communication is a necessity.

Start Small

Setting boundaries is a skill that takes a while to develop, especially if it's something you've never done before. Therefore, start with a small boundary, like no phone calls after a certain time at night. Make sure to follow through;

otherwise, the boundary is worthless. From here, make larger boundaries based on your comfort level.

Eliminating Toxicity and Not Caring About Losing Friends

If you plan on making self-care a priority in your life, I think that's great, and so should you. However, some people will have a problem with this. People don't always like it when their friends, family members, or acquaintances, etc., put themselves at the forefront of their lives. Once again, that is their problem, not yours. What is your problem, though, is distancing or even eliminating these individuals from your life. We will go over that in this section because part of self-care is eliminating toxicity from your life and not feeling bad about it.

Don't Expect People to Change

While everyone deserves a chance to redeem themselves, there comes the point where we must accept that people cannot change by force. They have to find it within themselves to make this change, and it is not our responsibility to do so. You may yearn to be the one who changes them, but it's usually a hopeless project. Toxic individuals are motivated by their problems. They use them to get the attention they need. Stop being the one to give it to them.

Establish and Maintain Boundaries

I already went in-depth on this, so I won't revisit it too much here. Just know that toxic people will push you to work harder and harder for them, while you completely ignore your own needs. This is exhausting and unacceptable. Create the boundaries you need with these individuals based on your own limits.

Don't Keep Falling for Crisis Situations

Toxic people will make you feel like they need you always because they are constantly in a crisis situation of some sort. It is a neverending cycle. When a person is in a perpetual crisis, it is of their own doing. They often create drama purposely to get extra attention. You may feel guilty for ignoring them, but remember that their being manipulative and not totally genuine.

I am not saying that you can't ever help someone who is going through a hard time. Of course, you can. Just don't start believing that you're responsible for their success or failure.

Focus on the Solution

Toxic individuals will give you a lot to be angry and sad about. If you focus on this, then you will just become miserable. You must focus on the solution, which, in this case, is removing drama and toxicity from your life. Recognize the fact that you will have less emotional stress once you remove this person from your life. If you let them, they will suck away all of your energy.

Accept Your Own Difficulties and Weaknesses

A toxic person will know how to exploit your weaknesses and use them against you. For example, if you are easy to guilt-trip, they will have you feel guilty every time you pull away from them. If you get to know yourself better and recognize these weaknesses, then you can better manage them and protect yourself. This goes along with creating self-awareness, which we discussed in chapter two. When you accept your weaknesses, you can work on fixing them and balance them with your strengths.

They Won't Go Easily

Recognize that a toxic individual may resist being removed from your life. Actually, if they don't resist, I will be pleasantly surprised. They may throw tantrums, but this is because they can't control or manipulate you anymore. They will even increase their previous tactics with more intensity. It is a trap, and you must not fall for it. Stay firm in your desire to leave and keep pushing forward. If they suck you back in, good luck trying to get out again.

Choose Your Battles Carefully

Fighting with a toxic person is exhausting and usually not worth it. You do not need to engage in every battle with them. They are just trying to instigate you.

Surround Yourself With Healthy relationships

Once you have removed a toxic person, or persons, from your life, then avoid falling into the trap with someone else. Fill your circle with happy and healthy relationships, so there is no room for any toxicity. Always remember the signs of a toxic person, so you can avoid them wholeheartedly in the future.

How to Focus on Self-Care

Now that we have worked to set boundaries and eliminate toxic people from our lives, it is time to focus on ourselves and the self-care we provide. The following are some self-care tips, according to psychologist, Dr. Tchiki Davis, Ph.D.

Pay Attention to Your Sleep

Sleep is an essential part of taking care of yourself. You must make it part of your routine because it will play a huge role in your emotional and physical well-being. There are many things that can wreak havoc on your sleep patterns, like stress, poor diet, watching television, or looking at your phone as you're trying to fall asleep. Think about your night routine. Are you eating right before bed or taking in a lot of sugar and caffeine? Are you working nonstop right up until bedtime? Have you given yourself some time to wind down before going to sleep? All of these factors are important to consider, as they will affect your sleep patterns. If you can, put away any phones, tablets, and turn off the television at least 30 minutes before you plan on going to bed.

Take Care of Your Gut

We often neglect our digestive tract, but it plays a major role in our health and overall well-being. When our gut is not working well, it makes us feel sluggish, bloated, and nonproductive. Pay attention to the food you eat as it will determine the health of your gut. It is best to avoid food with excess salt, sugar, cholesterol, or unhealthy fats. Stick to foods that are high in fiber, protein, healthy fats, and complex carbs. Some good options are whole grains, nuts, lean meats, fruits and vegetables, beans, and fish.

Exercise and Physical Activity Is Essential

Regular exercise is great for both physical and mental health. The physical benefits are obvious. However, many people do not realize that exercise will help the body release certain hormones like endorphins and serotonin. These are often called feel-good hormones because they play a major role in affecting our mood in a positive way. The release of these hormones will give us energy too, which will make us want to exercise more. Once exercise becomes a habit, it will be hard to break. Decide for yourself what your exercise routine will be, whether it's going to the gym, walking around the neighborhood, or playing a game of tennis.

Consider a Mediterranean Diet

While this is not a dietary book, the Mediterranean diet is considered the healthiest diet in the world because of its extreme health benefits. The food groups and ingredients that are used will increase energy, brain function, and has amazing benefits like heart and digestive tract health. The food also does not lack flavor, which shatters the myth that healthy food does not taste good.

Take a Self-Care Trip

Even if you are not much of a traveler, getting away once in a while can do wonders for your mental health. So often, our environment will make us feel stressed out, and it's good to remove ourselves from it for a couple of days. You do not have to take a trip abroad here. Of course, that is certainly an option. A simple weekend trip is perfectly fine. Just get yourself out of your normal routine and be by yourself for a while.

Get Outside

Nature and sunlight can be great medicines. It can help you reduce stress or worry, and has many great health benefits. Doing some physical activity outside, like hiking or gardening, are also great options.

Bring a Pet Into Your Life

Pets can bring you a lot of joy, and the responsibility they come with can boost your self-confidence by having to care for another living creature. Dogs are especially great at helping to reduce stress and anxiety. Animal therapy has been used to help people suffering from disorders lie PTSD, as well.

Get Yourself Organized

Organizing your life and doing some decluttering can do wonders for your mental and emotional health. Decide what area of your life needs to be organized. Do you need to clear your desk, clean out the fridge, or declutter your closet? Do you need to get a calendar or planner and schedule your life better? Whatever you can do to get yourself more organized, do it. Being organized allows you to know how to take better care of yourself.

Cook Yourself Meals At Home

People often neglect the benefits of a good home-cooked meal. They opt, instead, for fast-food or microwave dinners. These types of meals will make you full but will lack in essential nutrients that your body needs. Cooking nutritious meals at home will allow you to use the correct ingredients, so you can feel full and satisfied. Cooking alone can also be great therapy for people.

Read Regularly

Self-help books are a great read. However, do not limit yourself to these. You can also read books on subjects that you find fascinating or books that simply provide entertainment.

Schedule Your Self-Care Time

Just like you would write down an appointment time in your planner, also block out specific times for self-care activities. Stick to this schedule religiously, unless a true emergency comes up. This means that if a friend calls you to go out, you should respectfully decline their request and focus on yourself.

Chapter 4: How to Be Happy Being Alone

The final section of this book will focus on being alone and how to be happy about it. When you start engaging in self-care, you will also be spending much more time by yourself. A lot of people have a hard time dealing with this concept, especially if they're used to being around people all the time. However, for proper self-care, you have to be okay with being alone once in a while.

Accept Some Alone Time

The following are some tips to help you become happy with being alone. Soon, you will realize that your own company is the best kind.

Do Not Compare Yourself to Others

We are referring to your social life here. Do not compare to others, and do not feel like you must live as others do. If you do this, you may become jealous of a person's social circle or lifestyle. It is better to focus on yourself and what makes you happy. If you plan on spending significant time alone, then you cannot pay attention to what other people are doing.

Step Away From Social Media

If strolling through your social media page makes you feel left out, then take a step back and put it away for a while. During self-care moments, you are the focus, not what is happening with others online. Also, what people post on their pages is not always true. Many individuals have been known to exaggerate, or even flat-out lie on social media platforms. You may be feeling jealous or left out for no reason. Try banning yourself from social media for 24-48 hours, and see how it makes you feel.

Take a Break From Your Phone

Avoid making or receiving calls. Let the important people in your life know that you will be away from your phone for a while, so they don't worry. When you are alone, really try to be alone.

Allow Time for Your Mind to Wander

If you feel unusual about doing nothing, it is probably because you have not allowed yourself to be in this position for a while. Carve out a small amount of time where you stay away from TV, music, the internet, and even books. Use this time to just sit quietly with your thoughts. Find a comfortable spot to sit or lie down, then just let your mind wander and see where it takes you. This may seem strange the first time, but with practice, you will get used to the new freedom.

Take Yourself on a Date

You don't need to be with someone else to enjoy a night out on the town. Take a self-date and enjoy your own company for a while. Go to a movie by yourself, stop by a nice restaurant, or just go do an activity you enjoy. If you are not used to hanging out alone, give it some time and you will become more comfortable with it. Take yourself on that solo date.

Exercise

We have mentioned exercise and physical activity a lot, but that's because it has so many great benefits related to self-care. Exercising will uplift your mood, and make it more enjoyable to be by yourself. Those feel-good hormones will provide a lot of benefits during these times.

Take Advantage of the Perks of Being Alone

Some people have spent so much time with other people that they've forgotten the perks of being alone. There are many to consider. First of all, you do not have to ask anyone's permission to do anything; you will have more personal space, can enjoy the activities you want to do, and don't have to worry about upsetting anyone. If you want, you can even have a solo dance party in your living room, Tom Cruise style. There are many advantages to being alone, so use them.

Find a Creative Outlet

It is beneficial to use some of your alone time to work on something creative. This can be painting, sculpting, music, writing, or any other creative endeavors. In fact, you can get out the watercolors and start fingerpainting. Creativity will bring a lot of joy into your life. It will make you happier about being alone.

Take Time to Self-Reflect

Being alone will give you the opportunity to self-reflect on your life. You won't care so much about being alone when you are coming up with important answers to your life.

Make Plans for Your Future

Planning out your life for five or ten years down the line will give you something important to do, and something to look forward to. Alone time is the perfect opportunity to determine these plans.

Make Plans for Solo Outings

Plan your solo outings based on what you like to do, whether it's a farmer's market, hiking, riding your bike, or going camping alone. Mak plans that will excite you, and you will be taking care of yourself while also being okay alone.

There are numerous topics that we went over in this chapter, but they all relate back to one theme: Self-care. Always remember that to take proper care of yourself, you must consider the following ideas:

- Setting Boundaries
- Avoiding and ridding yourself of toxic people
- Focus on yourself and your needs
- Be okay with being alone

Focus on these areas, and you will be demanding your own self-care without ever apologizing for it.

www.ingramcontent.com/pod-product-compliance
Lightning Source LLC
Chambersburg PA
CBHW071734080526
44588CB00013B/2028